TIRED
BUT
WIRED

TIRED
BUT
WIRED

**THE ESSENTIAL SLEEP TOOLKIT:
HOW TO OVERCOME YOUR SLEEP PROBLEMS**

Dr Nerina Ramlakhan

Souvenir Press

First published in Great Britain in 2010 by Souvenir Press Ltd
43 Great Russell Street, London WC1B 3PD

ISBN 9780285638778

Typeset by M Rules
Printed and bound in Great Britain

To my beloved sister and guiding light.
Wherever you are.

CONTENTS

Author's Introduction   1

Part 1 Understanding Your Sleep   9

Chapter 1   Sleep in a Changing World   11
Chapter 2   What Happens When You Sleep?   29
Chapter 3   When Sleep Goes Wrong   47
Chapter 4   Sleep is Only One Way of
              Recovering Energy!   69
Chapter 5   Are You Ready to Take Control
              of Your Sleep?   80

Part 2 The Sleep Toolkit   93

Chapter 6   The Nuts and Bolts   96
Chapter 7   The Basic Tools   112
Chapter 8   Power Tools I – Optimal Breathing   129
Chapter 9   Power Tools II – Optimal Breathing
              in Action   142
Chapter 10   Power Tools III – Mind Power   160
Chapter 11   Power Tools IV – To Sleep Perchance
              to Dream   181
Chapter 12   Putting it all Together   197

Part 3 Taking Action   201

Chapter 13   Case Study – Karen B Learns
                 to Sleep Perfectly   202
Chapter 14   Frequently Asked Sleep Questions   209

The Toolkit Made Easy   224
Further Reading   228
Useful Information and Resources   232
Acknowledgements   237

INTRODUCTION

I am *passionate* about helping people to sleep.

I believe that when we sleep, something wondrous happens. Nature (or God, depending on your beliefs) has given us this amazing ability to retreat from the day into stillness and renew our energy on every level – physical, mental, emotional and spiritual.

But for many of us, sleep can go wrong and when this happens time and time again we begin to lose the ability to tap into the process that gives us our vitality, optimism and strength of spirit. Not being able to sleep can affect our health, morale, relationships, social and working lives.

I've been working with sleep problems for over fifteen years and the world has certainly changed a lot during this time. At the beginning of my career, as a research scientist, I worked in a laboratory with six other scientists. We shared two computers, one telephone and a fax machine and we thought we were busy! Not so long after this I left the world of academia, working in Health Screening in a clinic in the City of London where it seemed as if everyone and everything was going faster and faster to try to keep up with the accelerating pace of technology. This was when my physiologist's brain started to become curious about how we modern day 'hunter-gatherers' were going to be able to adapt to our crazy 21st Century world . . . This was also when I noticed that increasingly my clients were coming to me with their sleep problems and fatigue.

Insomnia is a major public health problem. Every year, millions of pounds are spent on sleep medications – both prescribed and over-the-counter. The statistics indicate that one in ten adults has problems sleeping – I believe this underestimates the problem. Insomnia is one of the most common complaints encountered by doctors yet our medical profession struggles to find effective solutions and the most common recommendation is to prescribe sleeping pills.

But my interest in sleep isn't just academic or professional. It's also deeply personal.

My Story

My fascination with sleep began long before the years studying physiology and psychology at university, and well before the years spent in a clinic talking to hundreds of sleep-deprived City professionals. Maybe the fascination started when, as a young child growing up in a wooden-floored house in Guyana, I could hear my father pacing about at night, restless and unable to sleep. But perhaps my real interest stems from my own sleep problems which began when I was a teenager and lasted into my 30s. There were times when I felt I just didn't need it *at all* and other times when I felt absolutely exhausted but I just couldn't switch my brain off and go to sleep. In 1995 I hit rock bottom and became very ill and this marked the beginning of a long, slow and painful journey back to recovery.

During this process of recovery, I learnt how to sleep again. In fact, I learnt how to sleep *brilliantly* – but the story didn't end there. By a bizarre twist of fate I found myself working more and more with people's sleep problems and seeming to have the knack of sorting them out. In 2007 I joined the Capio Nightingale Hospital – a private psychiatric hospital in London – to run their sleep and energy programmes. My work now brings me in touch with stressed-out City executives, exhausted mothers and even elite athletes and I never tire of trying to sort out the huge range of sleep problems that I regularly encounter in my practice as well as trying to find effective solutions for them.

I now know that all of these experiences – even the most painful ones – created the foundations of how I have been able to help myself and then the exhausted clients who come to talk to me about their own sleep problems.

New Skills Needed

At the time of writing this book, I've never been busier. Sleep problems are on the rise and, in the last year, with the collapse of the financial markets and global crisis, I've seen a rising level of sleep problems coupled with fear and anxiety over the future. The irony is that I'm so busy that in order for me to be able to write my book, I've had to sacrifice some of my sleep! And this is the reality for many of us – we are so busy and it's impossible to 'expand' time and find more hours in which to get more sleep to fuel the demand. So we need to start thinking more creatively and intelligently about our energy and resilience. How can we ensure that the sleep we are getting is sufficiently deep and nourishing to meet this demand? Can we find ways other than sleep by which we can restore and renew our energy?

As technology continues to develop, we as human beings find ourselves going at full capacity. We need new ways of working, being and restoring our energy. *Our current practices are not sustainable.*

Tired but Wired isn't just about going to bed with rush hour traffic in your brain. It's also for those of you who have other sleep problems or just want more energy to live your life more fulfillingly. It's even for those of you who are incredibly blessed and *don't* have sleep problems and can sleep anytime and anywhere even if only so that you understand and can soothe the ruffled feathers of your tired and disgruntled bedmates.

How to use this book

I've set out to make this book as practical and accessible as possible. I will occasionally describe some scientific concepts that may help you to understand why you are experiencing problems with your sleep but this is absolutely **not** a scientific or medical textbook. I also hope to make these concepts as memorable as possible by telling you some real-life stories that I'm sure you will be able to relate to. Naturally, the names have been changed to protect the confidentiality of my clients but I promise you, these are real stories and I hope that you will feel less alone when you read them.

You will find this book laid out in three parts that cover the key elements of my sleep programmes:

- Part One: Understanding your sleep
- Part Two: The Sleep Toolkit
- Part Three: An in depth case study and Frequently Asked Questions chapter

Part One will help you to understand your sleep better – what happens when you sleep, and why it goes wrong. I'll ask you to think hard about whether you really are ready to take on the challenge of working on your sleep? – this is absolutely key to achieving the results you want.

In Part Two, The Sleep Toolkit, you'll find the tools that will really help you to create your unique version of sleep. After years of experimenting with my own sleep, studying sleep problems and helping my clients with their problems, I've amassed a collection of sleep tools. As I applied these tools to solving different sleep issues, I noticed that they could be grouped into different categories – some are very easy to use and can produce good results almost overnight for some of my clients. Others may take a little more effort and eventually produce very powerful returns. Although I originally started out as a research scientist I have learnt that there is a whole other part of my brain that gets involved in trying to help those who come to me with their sleep problems. Call it intuition or just plain experience. Whatever it is, the basis of my Sleep Toolkit isn't just grounded in hard science but also in an inner sense about sleep that I hope to impart to you throughout this book.

Part Three contains various pieces of additional information that I hope you will find helpful. Here I've included a Frequently Asked Questions section that you can use as a quick reference to solve your particular sleep problem. I'll also share with you a fascinating case study that beautifully demonstrates how the Sleep Toolkit can be put to use with amazing results.

For those of you who might be wondering 'what next?' the Further Resources section offers you some ideas of where to go for further help and support.

You don't have to read this book from cover to cover. If you're really sleep-deprived and desperate for some solutions, you might want to skip Part One and go straight through to the Sleep Toolkit. But I would encourage you to take the time to read the earlier sections of the book. Not only do they bring life and context to the mysterious and beautiful process of sleep but most importantly, I've found that when my clients begin to understand what is happening with their sleep, they are in a better position to take control of it and select the tools that work for them. Learning more may also offer you reassurance and sometimes my clients don't need to see me again after I've helped them to understand what is going on with their sleep.

Small Changes, Big Results

Some of the people who come to see me are very exhausted and for them, making big changes is inconceivable. Often it is the small changes that I encourage them to make that produce a big shift and set them on the right path to brilliant sleep. So take heart and don't be overwhelmed by what you think may lie ahead. *Small changes really can make a big difference.*

My Deepest Intention

I hope you will enjoy reading and learning about your sleep, but my intentions are far deeper than that. I hope you will benefit in at least **three** ways:

- **Better sleep** (of course) – My first aim is to get you the deep, peaceful, nourishing sleep that you deserve;
- **More energy** – my work continues to bring me in contact with hundreds of people every week and I see not just sleepiness but tiredness, fatigue, exhaustion and burnout. In these chapters you will learn not just about your sleep but also how to have the energy and vitality to live your life in the way you really want to;
- **Safety and equilibrium** – Feeling safe is a basic, essential and primitive need for every human being and one that we particularly need in these unusual and challenging

times. I believe that when we sleep we return to a place of 'safety' that restores on every level – physical, emotional, mental and spiritual. For many, when the connection with good sleep is broken this is experienced as the deepest disequilibrium possible – that of 'un-safety'. I hope that the tools I will share with you will help you to build an *inner core of safety* that is with you even during difficult and adverse times.

Although I can't truly replicate the quality of the interaction that would take place if you were sitting with me, I'm hoping that my energy and my intention will reach across to you in my words and that, like my clients and patients, you too will experience a beautiful reconnection with your sleep and vitality.

Read on, enjoy and I wish you brilliant sleep!

Part One

UNDERSTANDING YOUR SLEEP

Understanding more about *your* sleep will help you to take big steps towards sleeping well and feeling more energised. So I hope you won't be tempted to skip this part and move straight through to the toolkit as these chapters will provide a solid foundation to understanding your sleep and solving your sleep problems.

In this section you will see that we are actually designed to sleep well – I hope you will take reassurance from this. Then we will look at the process of sleep, what happens when we sleep and the purpose of the sleep stages and cycles, and why sleep goes wrong. You will also learn more about your energy and how to look after yourself more holistically so that you not only feel more vital and well, but you also sleep better.

CHAPTER 1

Sleep in a Changing World

How did you sleep last night?

Did you slide effortlessly into a cocoon of thick, velvety sleep? Did you awaken filled with energy and enthusiasm, looking forward to the day ahead?

Or did you crash out exhausted and then find you just couldn't sleep?

Are you Tired but Wired?

This book is about helping you to get brilliant sleep and by this I mean sleep that is deep, nourishing, refreshing and peaceful – sleep that is the opposite of Tired but Wired. I firmly believe that our physiology is actually designed to give us this type of sleep. In other words:

Your physiology is designed to give you brilliant sleep.

You may not believe this if you haven't slept well for a while and, in fact, you may even have forgotten what good sleep feels like. But somewhere along the line, something has disrupted the natural process of your sleep and brilliant sleep is for you either a distant memory or something you have *never* had.

How can something that is so natural, so innate and actually *hardwired* into our physiology go so wrong for some of us? There are many factors that can disrupt sleep – and you will learn more about this as you read further. But I believe that there is something about our 21st Century world that has had a particularly significant impact on our sleep and the ability to renew our energy.

Faster and Faster

At the time of writing, I've never been busier – juggling writing, professional commitments, time for my family and friends, time to look after myself and time to sleep. But I'm not alone in this – everywhere I go I see the same pressurised busyness and *go, go, go!*

The world we are living in is going faster and faster driven by technology and globalisation. We struggle to keep up and find ourselves reaching for caffeine, energy drinks, anything that will help us to fuel the manic need to do more and in less time. For many of us in the Western world our days are relentlessly linear, we rarely go 'offline'. The word 'downtime', originally used to describe the cessation of operations in a manufacturing or engineering environment, is now used to describe the guilt-ridden periods of rest that increasingly we have less time for. At night we retire to bed desperate for some rest and then find we just can't relax, we just can't stop and *be*.

I began using the phrase Tired But Wired firstly to describe my own sleep and then that of my clients and patients. For many years, I went to bed with crazy snippets of conversations

I'd had throughout the day, music I'd listened to and random to-do lists, all playing at extra loud volume in my brain. It was driving me mad and stopping me from sleeping – even if I was exhausted. I never questioned it. It was just me, wasn't it? And then I started working in a clinic and seeing stressed out bankers, teachers, lawyers, over-stretched mothers, and even anxious school children and noticed that they would describe the same 'noise' to me.

At the same time, the pace of technology had taken off and everyone seemed to be grappling with the same challenges of information overload, and trying to fit even more into their lives. It seemed the treadmill had stepped up a few notches and this played havoc with my clients' energy levels and, in particular, sleep. When I used the phrase Tired but Wired I would see an immediate look of comprehension and relief on their faces. 'At last! Someone who understands.'

Technology – Friend or Foe?

Don't get me wrong – I'm definitely not a technophobe. I love the fact that I can press a few buttons and in the blink of an eye, my parents who are thousands of miles away will see the most recent image of their 5yr old granddaughter. I love the fact that browsing the Internet has saved me hours of precious time that would have been spent getting to a library and then finding the material that I needed to write this book. I'm amazed by the fact that in realtime using Webcasts and Webinars, I can get my message out to thousands of people living in a different time zone. Technology is amazing!

But I'm also sadly aware that something is slipping away from us . . . In this millennium we increasingly see relationships that are managed by text messages or in chatrooms, school children who have forgotten the art of reading or creating their own stories as they lift paragraphs of easily accessible homework from the Internet. We hear about more and more problems that have arisen as a result of using, or rather abusing, technology. At the hospital we see young people suffering from technology addiction, people complaining of loneliness because of the lack of real human connection, and people suffering from Tired but Wired and insomnia.

The fundamental flaw in all of this is that we as human beings haven't quite caught up with technology. As James Gleick says in his book *Faster*, we are reaching *'the biological, psychological and neurological limits of just how much we are capable of doing.'*

The Pulse of Life

Human beings are not meant to be relentlessly linear – we are meant to oscillate moving rhythmically between energy expenditure (work) and energy renewal (recovery and renewal). In the 19th Century Claude Bernard was the physiologist who was responsible for a major breakthrough in the understanding of how living organisms remain in a state of balance and equilibrium despite fluctuations in our external environment. He called this **homeostasis**, which is described as the maintenance of a constant internal environment that is essential for survival. What this means is that living organisms make small internal adjustments – oscillations – to maintain an internal state of balance and equilibrium. For example, in response to eating a piece of delicious chocolate your blood sugar rises. To stop the level of sugar in the blood from reaching critical limits (and damaging the brain), the pancreas produces insulin that carries the sugar away for storage thus causing a fall in blood sugar. So the rise in the sugar level in the blood triggers reactions that then cause a subsequent fall. Thus your blood sugar hovers around an equilibrium point. This oscillation process is vital for your health and when it stops working normally – for example in diabetes – you become ill.

Many years ago, I noticed that whenever I talked to my clients or students about the control of body temperature, stress, appetite, breathing, in fact, any physiological process, I would draw an oscillating curve that went up and then down. I went on to use this as a symbol for my business 'Equilibrium Solutions' as I began to realise that every technique I taught was focused on creating balance or a constant internal state. I also noticed that the 'oscillating line' was particularly relevant to sleep.

The big oscillation of the day is the **circadian rhythm** or 24hr cycle. This means that within a 24hr phase we are awake and active and then, as the light drops, we rest and sleep.

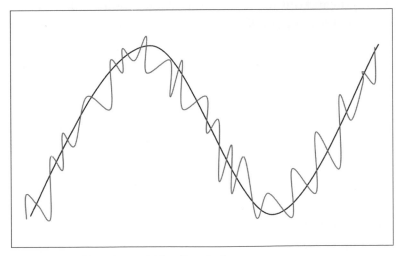

Figure 1: The Circadian and Ultradian rhythms

However, built into this 24hr cycle – and this is where I believe Tired but Wired has its roots – is a shorter cycle of about 90 minutes. This is called the **ultradian rhythm.** This is the pulse or 'hum' of our energy as we go through the day – our basic rest/activity cycle. And the relevance of this shorter cycle? It means that we are designed to renew our energy throughout the day, build pauses into our day, stop, rest and then go again. We are meant to build oscillation into our day. When we don't, we accumulate fatigue and the sleep process itself becomes disrupted as it tries to overcorrect the imbalance that has been created during the day.

In the Western world, we have simply lost the art of stopping – and it really is as simple as that. Ten to fifteen years ago I worked in organisations where it was normal for people to stop for a tea or coffee break for 15 minutes or so. We stopped and had lunch. We stopped working when we went home and we certainly didn't work on the way home. In today's world it has become harder and harder to stop. There's always something else to do and this relentless drive to keep 'doing' takes us further and further away from the ultimate form of rest – that of sleep.

I recently worked with Ben, a very successful lawyer who was suffering from insomnia. He came in to see me clutching his mobile phone which he glanced at constantly during our session. He said, 'I'm good at thinking. I'm paid to think and I love thinking. The problem is that I can't stop thinking when I get into bed at night and it's driving me mad. I have to get up around 3am to work because I just can't switch my brain off. My day is relentless and at night I need to get some sleep!' My work with Ben was short and sweet and mainly involved getting him to set some rules about when he switched his phone off – particularly at home in the evenings. Initially, he was sceptical that such a small change could make such a big difference. After two weeks of developing a healthier relationship with his mobile phone, Ben's sleep was not only more peaceful and restorative, but he woke in the mornings feeling energised and looking forward to the day ahead.

The Return to Sleep

When we sleep – and in order for us to be able to sleep – we return to a child-like state of trust, acceptance, and softness. We let go of worries and anxieties. We relinquish control and needing things to be *just so.*

But for many the stress of life means it becomes impossible to let go and stop trying. Throughout the day we become more and more tightly coiled, trying harder, not letting go, and at night this softness, trust and acceptance is simply inaccessible. Some people are so tightly coiled it is as if they are actually 'working' all night not just mentally (thinking all night) but physically (restless, jerking and twitching). Not surprisingly, they wake up exhausted and with aches and knots that have developed while they slept.

When I work with my clients, my **greatest** intention is to move them closer to this state of letting go and softness – because this is when they will sleep. I do this by using techniques and tools that I will be sharing with you very soon but for now, I would like to tell you a little about how I arrived at using these tools.

If we search with sufficient persistence, we will nearly always find an evolutionary explanation for human behaviour. After all, all human physiology and behaviour can be attributed to the process of evolution. So is it possible that the way we slept so many years ago can offer some solutions to the sleep challenges we face today? The answer to this question is a resounding 'yes!' and this belief is borne from the work I have done with my own sleep and my work with thousands of sleep-challenged individuals.

Let's take a brief journey back in time . . .

Sleep in an Unsafe World

It was a blazing hot morning. The sun rose in the sky and with it rose the temperature. The hunters longed to stop and seek shelter from the burning heat but they couldn't. Food and water were scarce. They had been hunting for more than three days – running, walking, stumbling across rough terrain – and though they needed to stop and rest, this simply was not possible. They desperately needed to replace the fuel that their activity had burned away.

Once upon a time, thousands of years ago, our world wasn't quite as it is today: climatic conditions were harsh, food was scarce and the environment was rife with predators. Maybe there would have been times when it simply wasn't safe enough to sleep – we needed to stay awake to hunt and gather food, or to ward off predators. Of course if all was well in our world, we slept as the sun went down and woke when the sun rose. But some of the time *sleeping simply wouldn't have been convenient or conducive to our survival.*

SO HOW IS THIS RELEVANT TO SLEEPING IN THE 21ST CENTURY?

Well in many respects we are still cavemen (and women). It takes thousands of years to change your genetic code – the DNA that contains the blueprint or recipe for every aspect of your biological functioning. Although neuroscientists have yet to discover a specific 'sleep gene', it is still possible that the 'sleep formula' of a primitive hunter-gatherer is still encoded somewhere in your sleep pattern!

Many years ago when I began helping people with their sleep problems, it became very apparent to me that there were elements of our ancestral sleep programming that were not only relevant to how we sleep in the 21st Century but incredibly important in helping to restore and create the brilliant sleep that we all crave.

Back to the Future

It is not the strongest of the species that survives, nor the most intelligent, but the one most responsive to change.
— Charles Darwin

By going 'back to the future' I have come up with **four key elements** that form the core of my sleep programmes and these are:

1. **Rest** is the essential precursor to brilliant sleep;
2. **Flexibility** creates brilliant sleep;
3. **Resourcefulness** — we are far more resourceful than we think and sleep is only one way of renewing our energy;
4. **Safety** is strongly linked to sleep;

The Rest-Sleep Connection

I have said there may have been a time when human beings slept very little and sleep was a luxury. So what did we do? Well we *rested* — whenever we could. We rested to build up our energy for hunting and gathering and to maintain our wellbeing and this would have had to be enough. And then, as we evolved and became better at protecting ourselves, building shelter, and foraging more efficiently, the intensity of our rest periods became more intense and we slept. Again, it may not have been conducive to our safety and survival to pass out for hours at a time and sleep, so throughout the day we slept or rested in short phases, whenever we could.

In other words, *rest was the substitute for sleep.*

So how have I used this information in my sleep programmes? Early on in my work I realised that a key to getting my patients to sleep was to 'go back in time' and teach them how to rest properly! This might sound obvious but, as I have said before, for so many people rest is a distant memory – the thing that you do at the end of the day, at the weekend, when you go on holiday. Or as one of my more cynical clients said 'when I die'!

The problem with living so rest-lessly is that it's almost like a muscle memory – when the body forgets how to rest it forgets how to sleep. This may help you to understand why even though you may have been going at full tilt all day (and therefore should be tired enough to sleep) you get exactly the opposite – Tired but Wired! In my sleep programmes, I show my clients exactly how and when to rest so that sleep becomes less of a distant memory. In fact, this is one of the ways in which my work differs from many other sleep programmes in which sleep-deprived patients are told that they *absolutely must not* sleep or rest during the day in order to be tired enough to sleep at night. Now this may be the case for some sleep problems, but often I will teach my clients how to start *attuning themselves to rest during the day so that their bodies are ready to accept sleep at night.*

What do I mean by 'rest'? I'm often asked this question. Don't worry, when we get to the Sleep Toolkit in Part 2 I'll show you exactly how to rest, but now, because this is such an important part of the programme, I would like to illustrate what I mean by sharing my neighbour Brian's story.

Brian was having some problems with his sleep – his main problem was that he was so tired in the evening that he would fall asleep in front of the TV, often sleeping for one or two hours, he would miss his favourite programmes and then find he couldn't sleep when he dragged himself to bed. As a director in a telecommunications company he was extremely busy, working long hours with very few breaks in the day. Each day, he drove to and from work while listening to the news on his radio. Brian's day was filled with information; his day totally lacked oscillation and his working memory was in overdrive. In the evening, when he finally stopped, his brain immediately went 'offline' and he fell asleep.

I wanted to help my neighbour so I suggested he start building some downtime into his day. I mentioned the word 'lunch break'. 'Oh, I do take a break,' he said, 'I just muck around on the Internet for half an hour or so while I eat.' So of course I told him about breaks and the working memory. He immediately decided to change his lunchtime routine and maybe even go for a walk sometimes. He sometimes even has a 15-minute power nap in the afternoon. Brian has stopped falling asleep in front of the TV in the evening.

Simply, rest can be defined as passive or active. The most important aspect of your rest break is that you do something unrelated to stimulation and information and that you give your brain the chance to go offline.

ACTIVE REST	PASSIVE REST
fast walking	practising a relaxation technique
jogging	powernapping
doing sudoku	listening to music
doing a crossword	meditation and prayer
eating a healthy snack	visualisation techniques

Active and Passive Rest

Sleep flexibility

This is the label that I use to describe that fact that we possess an innate ability to deviate from the 'normal' pattern of sleeping

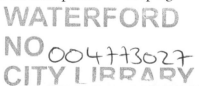

at the end of the day and this ability can have big advantages. So where does this ability come from? There is evidence that the early hunter-gatherers slept in short bursts of time throughout the day as *it would not have been conducive to their safety and survival to have retired into our caves at the end of the day and slept for 7 or 8 hours at a stretch.*

This marked the development of the human *polyphasic* sleep pattern in which there are several (poly) phases of sleep in a 24-hour period.

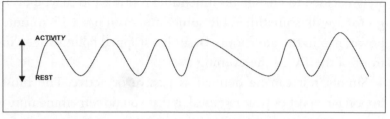

Figure 2: A polyphasic sleep pattern in which there are several periods of rest/sleep in a 24hr period.

WHERE ELSE MIGHT YOU SEE THIS SORT OF SLEEP PATTERN?

Of course our pets and babies and children! In fact, when my daughter was born she seemed to sleep most of the day and occasionally woke to play for a while, to have her nappy changed and to be fed. As she grew older, she started to lose her naps until most of her sleeping was happening at night. Now, at the age of five she very occasionally needs a short nap in the afternoon but generally does all of her sleeping at night. If she sleeps during the day, she needs less sleep at night and delays going to bed. She now has a fully, evolved *monophasic sleep pattern* in which she needs just one main sleep phase at night.

At the time of writing this, my husband, a police officer, has returned from working a night shift. Last night he began work at 10pm, completed his shift at 7am and will now sleep until the early afternoon. He is following a monophasic sleep pattern but has shifted it around to meet the demands of his job.

In 2002, Ellen MacArthur competed in the Vendee Globe in which she set a new world record for fastest circumnavigation of the globe as a solo sailor. During this race, which lasted 72 days, she had 385 naps and her longest period of sleep lasted 35 minutes. MacArthur learned how to do this by working with Dr Claudio Stampi, a leading sleep scientist, who taught her techniques (which you will learn later in the book) of napping so that she could recoup her energy throughout the race without needing to sleep for long periods of time.

Stampi's research has led to theories that humans have been polyphasic nappers for thousands of years before adopting our current monophasic pattern. In fact, it was Stampi's work that showed that even within the 24hr daily circadian cycle, we have the 'mini' activity/rest cycles of 90 minutes or so – the ultradian cycles I mentioned before.

So what does all of this mean and how is it relevant to our sleep today?

Well the most important thing is that we have the potential to be incredibly adaptable and flexible towards our sleep. In fact, even today in some traditional hunter-gatherer tribes such as the !Kung of Botswana and the Efe of Zaire sleep is a very fluid process: they sleep when they feel like it – during the day, in the evening, in the dead of the night. And of course, you will have heard of the Mediterranean types who have the very civilised habit of having an afternoon siesta.

Now I am not recommending that you start radically changing your sleep patterns and habits and if you are suffering with insomnia or other sleep problems – this may be the last thing you should be contemplating doing. However, an important part of my work is to encourage my patients to start cultivating more flexibility towards their sleep, to let go of inflexible and unhelpful beliefs. When they do this, time and time again I see something magical happen and they start to sleep like a baby . . .

Resourcefulness

Going back to the days of the caveman, we would probably have become an extinct species if we *absolutely needed* 7 or 8 hours of pure, uninterrupted sleep in order to be able to function efficiently the next day! So flexibility was key to our survival but also, we are very resourceful and *sleep is only one way in which we recover energy.* I am sure there are times when you have slept badly – the night before an exam, big presentation or before getting up early to go on holiday – but somehow, the next day you feel fine. So in my work I encourage my clients to really think holistically about their energy and we pay attention to nutrition, movement, hydration and even their mental, emotional and spiritual habits. By doing this, it takes the pressure off their sleep and ironically, they end up feeling more energised and *sleeping better.* Naturally, I will be sharing this holistic approach with you in my Sleep Toolkit.

Safety and sleep

Just for a moment let's return again to the hunter-gatherer and his cave. Before he retired to sleep on his mat of leaves he would have had to make an assessment of the situation. Is anything going on out there in the world that might threaten the existence of my family and me?

IN OTHER WORDS, IS IT SAFE ENOUGH FOR ME TO SLEEP?

So for every human being, *there is a very basic and primitive need to feel safe and secure before we can sleep.*

And we're not alone in this. Every animal needs to feel safe in order to rest and sleep. Think about your pets – don't they have their favourite sleeping places? Their own special routines and rituals that they adopt before they will sleep? I remember the trouble that ensued when I once replaced my cat's smelly basket with a brand new fluffy one – for two whole weeks she refused to go anywhere near it and just sat glaring at it (and me) accusingly. In the end, it took a lot of bribery, stroking and treats before she would accept it as her new bed!

I've noticed recently that 'safety' has become a major issue for many of my clients and it is this issue that is stopping them sleeping. Much of this is to do with the collapse of the financial markets and the 'credit crunch'. Many of them have uncertainties about the future and financial security. Some of the techniques that you will learn about in the Sleep Toolkit are not only designed to help you sleep better but also to develop an *inner core of safety* that remains strong even during adverse times.

So now you know a little about my sleep programme and the theory behind it. Allow me to bring this theory to life by sharing with you one of my favourite success stories.

Shona – The Journalist

When Shona came to see me she was exhausted and sleep-deprived. She said, 'I've never been a great sleeper but it's gotten particularly bad in the past 18 months. Two years ago there was a fire in my flat while I was sleeping. Luckily I wasn't hurt but it was a huge shock to be woken at 3am with the smoke alarms ringing. I now have problems getting to sleep and I wake every morning at 3am and can't get back to sleep. The worst thing is I'm exhausted but I just can't switch my brain off and I *really* need at least 7 hours of sleep to function normally the next day.'

Clearly the traumatic event of the fire had left some lasting and disturbing impressions but Shona also had some habits and beliefs that were making the problem worse. As a busy journalist she was on the go all day long. She spent hours in front of her computer and at night, even worked in bed on her laptop. During the night she phoned and text messaged friends from her BlackBerry that was left switched on beside her as she tried to sleep. To help her get to sleep she watched TV in bed as she drifted off to sleep, waking an hour or so later to switch it off. She then struggled on and off to sleep all night, checking the clock each time she awoke and worrying about how she was going to cope the next day.

SO HOW DID I WORK WITH SHONA?

Well first of all I got her to look at her day and whether there was any **rest** or oscillation built into it. I set her the task of taking more breaks from her computer and to actually move more every 90mins or so to break up the routine of sitting at her desk for hours. I taught her a 15-minute power napping technique that she used in the afternoon whenever she could to recoup some energy and attune her body to rest.

Next we worked on **flexibility** and **resourcefulness** . . . I asked Shona to consider that she could actually cope if she didn't get her 7 hours of sleep. Even though she wasn't entirely convinced by this she would say to herself, 'it doesn't matter if I don't sleep for 7 hours tonight, I'll still be fine tomorrow'. She also noticed that sometimes even a 10 minute power nap in the afternoon was enough to help her re-energise which got her thinking and behaving more flexibly towards her sleep. Following the principle of **resourcefulness** we looked at how she was looking after herself – her eating patterns, caffeine intake, and exercise habits – thereby taking some of the pressure off her sleep.

Finally, there was a lot to be done around **safety** and we started with the easy things. Shona had very few boundaries when it came to her work and her bedroom was filled with reminders of work that needed to be done. In a strange way, this was fuelling the feeling of 'it's not safe to sleep'. So I got her to remove anything related to work from her bedroom and set her the task of working on her time management – she started keeping organised lists. Shona stopped watching TV in bed and instead chose to read a carefully selected book that was light, funny and uplifting. She switched her mobile phone off early in the evening and left it in another room. She started keeping a journal that she wrote in whenever she felt stressed or overwhelmed. I taught her some yoga and relaxation techniques that she practised for 5 to 10 minutes before getting into bed at night. I asked her to stop checking the clock each time she woke up and taught her a breathing and visualisation technique to help her to return to sleep if she woke up in the night.

I saw Shona for three sessions and when I contacted her a year later to find out how she was getting on she was sleeping well and feeling great.

I will be sharing more stories with you throughout my book. I hope that by doing so you will not only feel less alone but will also begin to understand exactly what has gone wrong with your sleep and most importantly, how to put it right.

REMEMBER:

- We are physiologically wired for optimal sleep.
- Human beings are meant to oscillate between energy expenditure and renewal throughout the day.
- This process of oscillation is key to how we maintain an internal state of balance and how we sleep.
- We sleep well when we live our lives more restfully.
- Good sleep becomes possible when we can view our sleep more flexibly.
- We are very resourceful and sleep is only one way in which we recover our energy. Paying attention to other aspects of our energy takes the pressure off our sleep and helps to create brilliant sleep.
- We sleep well when we feel safe.

CHAPTER 2

What happens when you sleep?

I always tell my clients something about the process of sleep. Not only do I think it's fascinating but even my most exhausted and sleep-deprived clients wake up a little when I begin describing the science of sleep. But most importantly, I have found that helping clients to understand what is happening with their sleep moves them closer to taking control of it. It also dispels some of the unhelpful beliefs we might have about what we think constitutes good or bad sleep.

Why we sleep

We sleep 1/3 of our lives away.

– Albert Einstein

If it's true that we spend so much time asleep why is sleep so important? Surprisingly no one fully understands why we engage in this mysterious non-activity. In evolutionary terms it might seem that the semi-consciousness that comes with sleep is a risky proposition, one that makes us vulnerable as our ability to perceive our environment and to respond to any possible threat is reduced.

When we sleep most of our sensory input stops or slows down as do many of our physiological processes. We are unaware of ordinary sounds and close our eyes to eliminate visual input. Our nervous system slows our breathing, heartbeat and blood pressure. Waste production also lessens to prevent disruptions to our sleep. While our physiological functions are minimised, our brain too adjusts itself to reduced sensory input and operates on a very primitive level.

WHY DOES THIS HAPPEN?

Some scientific theories suggest that we sleep more for the brain than the body – that we sleep in order to process and file information that was taken in during the day and to repair and rebuild memory. Other theories place emphasis on the need for sleep to repair and grow the body physically; to keep the immune system robust and our physiological systems in perfect working order.

I believe that the process of sleeping does all of this and even more and when we sleep well the body is repaired and rebalanced physically, mentally, emotionally and even spiritually.

> *God bless the inventor of sleep, the cloak that covers all men's thoughts, the food that cures all hunger . . . the balancing weight that levels the shepherd with the king and the simple with the wise.*
>
> – Miguel de Cervantes *Don Quixote*

Here are just a few of the ways in which sleep repairs and rebalances our health:

Organisation of memory and consolidation of learning

Mood regulation

Immune system strengthening and repair

Nervous system growth and repair

Growth – many hormones that are vital for growth are timed
    for release during sleep

Your Sleep Architecture

When you sleep your body undergoes a number of complex
biochemical, hormonal and physiological changes. All of these
changes produce the sleep that is *unique to you*. Very shortly I
will describe what actually happens during the phases of sleep
but I don't want to give a bland impression of a process that is
identical in every human being. The structure and make up of
your sleep is unique to you and is what I call your *unique sleep
architecture*. In the previous chapter I said that your physiology
is designed to give you optimal sleep and this is the sleep that
is just right for you and keeps you well, vital and in balance. No
wonder we feel so bad when our sleep is disrupted.

SO WHAT ACTUALLY HAPPENS WHEN WE SLEEP?

When you sleep the levels of stress hormones that are produced
during the day drop off – adrenaline, noradrenaline and cortisol levels subside. This stress balancing effect of sleep is very
important and my clients who aren't sleeping well will often
complain of feeling anxious and panicky in the mornings. The
levels of growth and repair hormones start to increase – growth
hormone, prolactin, the sex hormones such as testosterone and
oestrogen. Levels of hormones and chemicals that are directly
involved in inducing and controlling the sleep cycles also
change: a chemical called adenosine increases throughout the

day as we expend energy. The levels of adenosine build up in the brain and cause sleepiness. Levels of serotonin (the feel-good hormone), melatonin and other chemicals such as tryptophan and dopamine also change.

I am sure that many of you will have heard that the hormone melatonin is important for your sleep. You may even have taken melatonin to help you sleep particularly if you have jet lag. Melatonin production is triggered by a signal from cells in the eyes (ganglions) indicating that light has fallen below ~200 lux. The role of melatonin is to communicate the pulse of the biological clock to every cell in the body – in other words it attunes the body to the circadian (24hr) cycle that I described previously. So melatonin production is dependent on darkness i.e. levels rise during the night and are suppressed by light. Melatonin is crucial for many biological processes but especially sleep and mood control.

Your nervous system also undergoes many changes while you sleep. Briefly, there is a large branch to your nervous system called the **Autonomic Nervous System (ANS) –** you will find out more about this when you get to the Toolkit and learn about some of the breathing techniques that will really improve your sleep. The ANS has two 'legs' to it – the **sympathetic nervous system (SNS)** and the **parasympathetic nervous system (PNS)**. It is this latter part of your nervous system, the PNS, that is *absolutely* key to you getting deep and peaceful sleep; when you activate the PNS it is thought to switch on those parts of the brain involved in initiating and maintaining your sleep.

The link between the brain and the PNS is via a nerve called the **vagus nerve**. The activation of this nerve is *crucial* to you being able to sleep. It is activated, quite simply, when you breathe from your diaphragm and when your breathing is deep and relaxed. In other words, when you are relaxed and your breathing is relaxed, you can sleep. It sounds so simple and it is simple but many of my clients are stressed and anxious and they *can't* relax or breathe deeply.

Many of my sleep tools are focused on activating the vagus nerve – they are simple, they work and I can't wait to share them with you!

The sympathetic nervous system, on the other hand, is the 'doing' part of our nervous system. It is what we need when we are busy and on the go. This part of the nervous system is also responsible for the production of adrenaline and other stress hormones that are produced when we are under threat – the so-called '**fight or flight**' response.

So in order for good deep sleep to occur

The parasympathtic nervous system needs to be active and fully engaged.

And

The sympathetic nervous system needs to be damped down and running at a very low level.

So you can see how Tired but Wired and bad sleep can be created by the wrong part of your nervous system being active, a sleep control centre that won't work and a disrupted internal sleep chemistry.

The Sleep Cycles

Now let's imagine you're feeling nicely relaxed and ready to sleep. Your breathing slows down and deepens, melatonin levels rise and your eyelids start to droop as you drift into the first phase of your sleep . . .

When we go to bed at night and wake up in the morning our sleep occurs in several stages. The ultradian cycle becomes more pronounced and we sleep in 90min cycles. The timing of these cycles is under the control of a process called the *circadian timer* – this influences when you sleep. When you travel across time zones, it is the disruption to this timer that causes jet lag. The pattern of our sleep is also controlled by a *sleep homeostat* that controls our 'drive' for sleep – so if you have been awake for a long time, the drive to sleep is increased to restore balance. You may remember that I referred to this in the previous chapter when I described the oscillation that is necessary to maintain our equilibrium and balance.

I sometimes compare the sleep control process to the central heating system in your house. Your heating may be triggered to switch on by two things: one is the timing you have pre-set (the circadian timer) and the other is the change in the temperature of your house (the sleep homeostat).

Figure 3 shows one 90-minute sleep stage and we might have three or four of these as we go through the night.

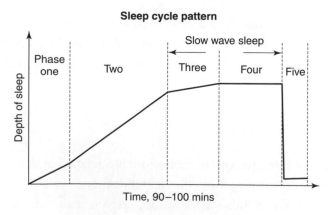

Figure 3: The Stages of Sleep

Each 90-minute stage of sleep is made up of four phases of **non-REM (rapid eye movement)** and **REM sleep**. The non-REM portion of sleep is phases 1 to 4. Phases 1 and 2 are **light sleep** and I often describe them as the 'warm up' for good deep sleep. 3 and 4 are slow wave or **deep sleep**. In phases 3 and 4, our brain wave activity slows down, and sleep deepens. This is what we experience as deep, nourishing, peaceful sleep. When we get enough of this kind of sleep we feel healthy, energised and physically and mentally well. We usually get this deepest sleep within the first hour of sleep – maybe it is nature's way of ensuring that we optimise badly needed sleep in case of external events prematurely interrupting our sleep.

At the end of each 90-minute stage comes the 10-15 minute burst of REM sleep. During this phase of sleep, our sleep depth becomes shallower and we can even drift into a state of semi-consciousness called a *hypnagogic trance*. We dream during this state and the brain cleverly deactivates our major muscle systems to stop us thrashing around, injuring ourselves and acting out our dreams. We may dream that we are running at top speed but our legs will only twitch. You can normally discern that someone is in REM sleep from the movements of the eyeball under the eyelid. There are theories that the brain takes us into the shallow states of REM sleep regularly throughout the night to prevent us from falling into a deep coma.

We also experience our first stage of REM sleep as we drift off into sleep – sometimes you get the sensation of falling or twitching. We usually experience a stage of REM sleep just before we wake up in the morning.

So throughout the night we cycle between non-REM deep sleep and REM shallow dreaming sleep and as we progress through the night the stage 4 deep sleep levels become more and more shallow. So effectively our deepest deep sleep occurs in the first sleep stage of the night.

So what function do these different stages serve?

REM Sleep

During REM sleep we experience two types of dreams:

1. 'Processing' dreams – for memory consolidation
2. 'Emotional' dreams – related to creativity, problem solving, trauma, emotional stress

Enter the Filing Clerk

Let's look at the first type of dreaming. During this type of dreaming we sort out information that we have handled recently so our dreams might be related to the conversations we have had, the bills, chores and to-do lists. We might even dream about the songs we have heard during the day. So during REM sleep, we undergo a very important tidying up and clearing out process. This is vital to our ability to learn and remember. I often say to my clients that during this stage of sleep, we invite a **filing clerk** into our heads to sort out our filing so that the next day we feel mentally sharp and clear.

The science of memory is highly complex and I am not going to go into this subject in any great depth – this is probably not what you are looking for if you are sleep-deprived. However, it is worth understanding a little about how our memory is organised and how I believe Tired but Wired can be created.

Memory has been divided into three categories based on how long the memory lasts:

The **sensory memory** – this acts as a repository for the
stimuli received by our senses, what we see, smell, touch,
hear. This site stores short-lived memories of milliseconds
to a few seconds.

The **working memory** – this stores memory for a little
longer but also processes information before passing on to
the third memory site.

The **long-term memory** – here information is stored from
anywhere between an hour to a lifetime.

So the working memory acts as a go-between for information we
are dealing with on a moment-by-moment basis and our long-
term memory. It is probably the most over-worked part of your
memory as you go about your day thinking, calculating, assessing,
remembering and communicating. The working memory is only
of finite size and can only hold limited information – I often
describe it as being similar to the inbox in your email system –
and it regularly recycles and frees up storage space in a few ways:

- when we go offline or simply stop and take a break
- when we daydream or even go into a trance-like state
- when we sleep

I believe that Tired But Wired arises when we reach the satu-
ration point of our working memory but try to work against
the natural cycle of going offline. So we reach for yet another
cup of coffee or we simply just keep going, running on will
power and adrenaline. The problem with this is that we then
start to accumulate a memory (and energy) debt and our com-
puting power or ability to concentrate or focus starts to drop.
Worst of all (from the point of view of sleep) is that it appears
that this memory debt that accumulates during the day inter-
feres with the memory consolidation process at night – either

we end up with too much 'work' to be done during our sleep or the 'filing' process becomes disrupted and disordered. Both of these feel like Tired but Wired sleep.

Anthropological research suggests that the working memory has evolved over millennia and that this has shaped the development of human beings from pre-modern *Homo Sapiens* to modern man and the age of computer technology. *However, I wonder if we have hit a wall in evolutionary terms and our brain and cognitive function, sophisticated as they may be, struggle to keep pace with technology and the rate at which we are able to process the information it throws at us?*

I believe that *this is where much of our* Tired But Wired *sleep can come from*. I believe that technology, and the resulting lack of 'downtime' has expanded our need for REM sleep that has given rise to this noisy, jangling, information-filled sleep that many of us complain of (and that has led you to my book).

Enter the Counsellor

The second type of dreams – what I call 'emotional dreams' – also occur during REM sleep. The invaluable function of such dreaming is to rebalance our emotions and sort out any traumatic memories but these rich dreams are also known for their problem-solving and creative functions.

It is well known that many important scientific discoveries were made during such dream states – Einstein's Theory of Relativity when he dreamt that he was riding on a beam of light or the German chemist Kekulé who was trying to determine the structure of benzene. He had been working on the supposition that benzene was a straight train molecule. One day, he fell asleep during a bus journey and during a hypnagogic dreamstate he dreamt of a chain of whirling atoms with the larger atoms curving back and dragging the smaller ones at the end of the chain. Thus he deduced that benzene is actually a ring structure.

This sort of dreaming feels very different from the 'processing' type of dreaming I have described above. Your dreams might be bizarre, nonsensical, symbolic and maybe even traumatic and upsetting. At the hospital, many of the patients who experience these types of dreams are creative types – artists, musicians, and writers. For some of them, it was the intensity of their dreams and an attempt to block them out that may have led them to addictions to alcohol and drugs. My work with such patients is often focused on getting them to 'befriend' their dreams and to see them as having the power to heal and solve their problems.

I often use the analogy that it is as if we have the best **counsellor** in our brain during this stage of sleep, sorting out our problems and healing our minds. Later you will learn exactly how to deal with such dreams if they are vivid, disturbing and affect your mood during the day.

There is so much that we still don't understand about why we dream but one thing that is clear is that we *all* dream and this process is vital for our emotional, mental and spiritual health. Even those of you who don't remember your dreams – just take some reassurance from knowing how much good work is going on while you sleep.

I believe that the increased need for 'processing' sleep may conflict with our ability to have the rich, symbolic, creative dreams that are so important for our sanity. In other words, the filing clerk and the counsellor are really up against each other.

Deep Sleep: Physical Renewal

During phases 3 and 4 of deep sleep we get the kind of sleep that really refreshes and rejuvenates the body – the kind of sleep that we all want. Levels of adrenaline, cortisol and other stress hormones start to drop and the brain starts to produce the hormones needed to repair the body. This is the sleep that keeps our immune systems robust, our skin looking fresh and unblemished, that gives us our sex drive and healthy digestion. Some people believe that deep sleep has almost magical properties. In Eastern philosophy, such sleep is referred to as *yogic* or *sattvic* (sanskrit for 'pure') sleep in which the body is renewed on every level – physical, emotional and spiritual.

So are we 21st Century sleep-deprived hunter-gatherers or are we just deprived of good, rejuvenating deep sleep?

I believe it is the latter.

Returning to our information-driven world, I believe that the increased demand for processing REM sleep compromises our deep sleep – in other words, we simply get less of it. We are probably getting more sleep than we've ever had in the history of mankind. Many of my patients at the sleep clinic are getting enough sleep in terms of actual hours (some of them are actually getting more than they realise but we will come to that later) but what they are falling short of getting is that rich and nourishing deep sleep. In the next chapter, you will learn more about how our sleep quality is affected by our lifestyle. Most importantly, in Part 2 you will go on to learn how to clean up and improve the quality of your sleep.

Sleep elasticity

Many people expect to go to bed and sleep *without waking* throughout the night. As I have mentioned earlier on, this is one of the most unhelpful expectations my clients have and one that I have to constantly challenge.

Do you remember waking up last night? And if so, how many times did you wake up? On average, a human being might wake an incredible 10 to 15 times a night! My clients are often astounded when I tell them this, as most of them (hopefully) will have no recollection of having woken so many times.

I call this *sleep elasticity* to describe the rebounding between sleep and wakefulness throughout the night. And why do we do this? One theory relates back to caveman days when it might have been helpful to maintain a state of vigilance even while we slept to avoid being eaten by predators.

If you don't remember waking several times last night, you are actually normal as technically, you haven't actually woken up but have drifted into a semi-conscious state. This is the trance-like *hypnagogic state* that I referred to earlier. In this state we assess safety, and drift effortlessly back into the next stage of sleep (figure 4).

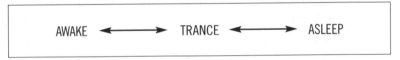

Figure 4: Sleep elasticity – rebounding between sleep and wakefulness.

When we enter the hypnagogic trance state, we gently touch semi-consciousness, rest there for a while, allowing ourselves to enjoy the delicious feeling of being warm, drowsy, safe, not awake and not asleep. Or at least, that is what should happen. For many, the return to sleep is the difficult part and the cycle back into sleep is broken.

Can we do without sleep?

I'm sure you would agree that sleep is not only complex but also an amazing process, but can we do without it? Sleep deprivation studies have been carried out to determine how little sleep human beings can get away with. The record for the longest period without sleep is 18 days, 21 hours, 40 minutes during a rocking chair marathon! However, the record holder reported hallucinations, paranoia, blurred vision, slurred speech and memory and concentration lapses.

So far the studies seem to indicate that we can't survive without sleep indefinitely. If you deprive someone of sleep by constant stimulation, they will eventually succumb to sleep and then will feel fully restored on waking, without any permanent damage.

I am often asked 'how much sleep do we need?' This varies from one person to the next and young people tend to need more than the elderly.

The work of Professor Jim Horne at the Sleep Research Centre in Loughborough and other workers has described two types of sleep: *core* sleep versus *optional* sleep. Core sleep is the first three sleep cycles (the initial 4-5 hours of sleep) necessary for human beings to function properly. Optional sleep is the 'nice to have' sleep that we can reasonably do without – again probably another 4 or 5 hours. However, there are large variations in how much sleep we need according to our stage of growth and development (see table below).

AGE RANGE	SLEEP REQUIREMENT
Newborn Baby	
Toddler	Up to 12hrs at night. 1–2 hrs during Day
By 4yrs	10–12hrs at night. No daytime nap.
Teenager	Approx. 9hrs but sleep timing can change
Adult	7–8 hours
Older adult	6–7 hours during day plus daytime naps

Average sleep requirements

To further complicate things, there is some evidence that there are some people who just need more sleep than others. Einstein being one of these such people. He apparently needed 10-11 hours of sleep particularly when he was working on something important. On the other hand, Margaret Thatcher famously only slept for five hours a night. Ernest Hartmann is a psychologist who has done some fascinating work looking at the personality differences between 'long' and 'short' sleepers. He found that long sleepers tend to be creative, more introverted, more emotional with complex personalities. By contrast, the shorter sleepers tended to be more contented and more socially adept. This theory is to be taken with a smallish pinch of salt – sleep is so complex and there are many reasons why people might over- or under-sleep. However, a particularly interesting feature of long sleepers' 'long' sleep is that they seem to experience twice as much REM sleep as the short sleepers – a strong indication that REM dreaming is needed for the processing of memories, creativity and the sorting out of our inner world.

There has also been some interesting debate recently about gender differences and sleep. Do women need more sleep than men or vice versa? Some studies suggest women need up to an hour extra sleep a night compared to men, and not getting it may be one reason women are much more susceptible to depression than men. In the week before menstruation many women feel they need more sleep as the demand for REM sleep increases during this stage of the menstrual cycle. There is also some fascinating research that shows that women's sleep elasticity can as much as double in the final trimester of pregnancy and for the first year or so of her baby's life. In other words, a new mother is likely to wake more times during the night than she did before having her baby. Furthermore – and this may settle a popular point of dispute between many new parents – *she does wake up more than the father* due to the birth-related changes in her sleep cycle. Perhaps this is an evolutionary mechanism that is essential for the survival of the baby?

The long and short of it is that sometimes we need more sleep than other times and the key is to start becoming more attuned to what we need. We also need to pay attention to all of the other vital aspects of our energy renewal – nutrition, hydration, movement, relationships, and even our spiritual health – thereby taking the pressure off sleep. You will learn more about energy renewal and your sleep very shortly.

Sleep Types

Now I know that I have said that your sleep is unique to you but some of us do show some similarities when it comes to timing of sleep.

Professor Jim Horne has developed a **larks** and **owls** theory. According to this theory, the body clock of some people is set for early rising – these are the so-called larks while owls tend to be late risers. Although both groups sleep roughly the same number of hours, the differences lie in the time of waking in the morning and the energy levels throughout the day. Larks find it easier to eat breakfast and can be the life and soul at breakfast time. On the other hand, owls can find it hard to get going in the morning, finding it difficult to stomach breakfast, can be somewhat grumpy. Larks are often the evening party poopers needing to cry off between 9 and 10pm while this is when the owls are well and truly in the swing of things!

However, these are extremes and in reality, most of us fall somewhere between the two. There is some small hereditary influence and age can also play its part: younger adults tend to be more owl-like and we become more lark-like with age. In general, owls tend to be more adaptable to enforced changes in their routines and body clock. I have done a lot of work with shift workers and have definitely found owls to be better at adapting to different work schedules than larks.

I have also come up with my own sleep types that are simply based on observations I have made with my clients over the years and which often bring instant looks of recognition when described. I have found that some people are what I call **Martini sleepers** – named after the famous cocktail from the 1980's – these individuals can sleep anytime, anyplace, anywhere! Often if people like this are attending my 'Sleep and Energy' group sessions at the hospital, they have come either because they are over-sleeping or their energy levels have hit rock bottom. On the other hand, there is another group that I call the **Sensitive sleepers**. If you are a sensitive sleeper you may have difficulty getting to sleep and things have to be *just so* in order for you to drop off. You are likely to wake at the slightest noise and then are more likely to have problems getting back to sleep.

Now I've worked with Martini sleepers who became sensitive sleepers and my work with them was about reconnecting them with the good sleep they once had – the advantage they have is that this good sleep is 'wired' into the memory and it's a question of trying to get it back.

On another positive note, Sensitive sleepers can become more Martini-like. I will cite myself as an example as I was once a very sensitive sleeper. I now sleep brilliantly most of the time and can even sleep on trains, planes and automobiles – something that was once impossible for me. For me, travel is now an invaluable opportunity not just to work and read but also to catch up on rest. However, if I am going through a particularly busy or stressful time, I do have to be mindful of using all of my sleep tools to maintain my good sleep. Once a sensitive sleeper, the tendency may always be there.

REMEMBER:

- All living organisms, including humans, run in cycles – long 24hr circadian cycles and short 90-minute ultradian cycles.
- These cycles govern our patterns of energy expenditure and renewal.
- We sleep in 90-minute cycles.
- Each sleep stage serves a different purpose – to file and process information and rebalance our physiology.
- It is normal to wake during the night and developing good sleep elasticity is key to creating good sleep.
- Our sleep is controlled by a complex interplay between the sleep control centre in the brain, hormones and chemical messengers and the nervous system.
- Brilliant sleep is dependent upon a balanced nervous system – a fully engaged parasympathetic nervous system and a reduced sympathetic nervous system.
- We can be categorised into different sleep types – owls and larks – depending on the preferred timing of our sleep.
- Some of us are more sensitive than others in our sleep habits and behaviours but can learn how to sleep wonderfully by applying the tools in Tired But Wired.

CHAPTER 3

When Sleep Goes Wrong

I love sleep. My life has this tendency to fall apart when I'm awake you know?

– Ernest Hemingway (1898-1961)

We *all* sleep badly from time to time.

There are some theories that we need the odd night of disrupted sleep to remind the body how to cope with the crisis of sleep lack and maybe to draw on other resources. Maybe it breaks the reliance on needing 6 to 8 hours of sleep in order to function – this makes sense in the light of what we have learnt about evolution and our sleep. Another theory about occasional bad sleep relates to the sleep homeostat you read about in the previous chapter when you learnt about the architecture of sleep. According to this theory, disrupted sleep kick-starts the sleep homeostat – almost like a tightening up of the screws in a machine – to maintain control of the sleep mechanism. In a way, this is the brain and body's way of reminding the sleep homeostat that it has a job to do and mustn't get complacent.

But when does the occasional bad night turn into chronic, debilitating insomnia and why does this happen? And what is insomnia?

What is insomnia?

The National Institutes of Health (NIH) in the USA defines insomnia as:

> *Complaints of disturbed sleep in the presence of adequate oppor-tunity and circumstances for sleep. The disturbances may consist of one or more of three features: (1) difficulty in initiating sleep, (2) difficulty in maintaining sleep, or (3) waking too early.*

Sleep clinicians also add to their list of diagnostic criteria the following:

How long the patient has had the problem
The impact on their life
How often it happens in a typical week
Its duration – how long does it take to get to sleep or resume sleep if you wake during the night?
The NIH also describes insomnia as sleeplessness lasting for more than a month.

As I've mentioned before, in my practice I work with those who are well but are having problems sleeping and at the hospital I see those who have become chronically ill and exhausted and their sleep problems may be severe. With this latter group, the sleep problem might end up causing a psychiatric problem or burnout (*primary insomnia*). On the other hand, their sleep problems may be part and parcel of a psychiatric problem such as anxiety or depression or even an addiction to drugs or alcohol (*secondary insomnia*). Sometimes it's difficult to unpick which came first – the sleep problem or the medical problems and/or psychological problems that subsequently arose.

The main problems I encounter in my practice with both groups are:

Problems getting to sleep (*sleep initiation*)
Problems staying asleep (*sleep maintenance*)
Waking too early
Oversleeping (*hypersomnia*)
Noisy, non-restorative sleep
Disturbing dreams
Teeth grinding

And then as a result of these sleep problems, my clients complain of tiredness and fatigue during the day, difficulty concentrating and finding the motivation to engage in anything. I often see people who have a mixed bag of sleep problems with combinations of the above. But what I see a lot of these days is what is called *paradoxical insomnia*. This is an odd one in which you may actually think you are *not* sleeping when in fact you are!

The first and most important thing I would like to say about insomnia is:

Insomnia isn't created at night.

Of course you become aware that you have a problem with sleep when you get into bed and then can't sleep. But this problem hasn't just been created in bed but rather has developed over the course of the day or even longer. I have clients who have had a lifetime of sleep problems some of which can be traced back to patterns and habits they have developed from childhood. Over time, these patterns and habits become hard-wired into their physiology eventually causing chronic sleep problems.

The Spiral into Insomnia

Yesterday in my clinic I saw a variety of people with sleep problems. One of them was a bright young female lawyer who I have worked with on and off for two years. She has suffered in the past from chronic fatigue and is now back at work and more or less, firing on all cylinders. Every now and then, when the pressure builds up at work and she has to work long hours, some of her old insomnia problems return and she has problems getting to sleep, she wakes in the early hours, finds it hard to return to sleep and then feels tired and irritable the next day. She comes to see me, we go over some basics, I offer reassurance and she is able to correct the imbalance in her sleep relatively easily. The 'mini' bout of insomnia passes.

Later in the day I saw a talented jazz musician who has had a lifelong history of sleep problems – he has always had problems getting to sleep and more recently, with the breakup of his marriage, his problems have worsened. He is also an alcoholic and for years has been using alcohol to pass out every night.

My last client of the day was Paul, a 40yr old night shift worker who has never had any sleep problems until 3yrs ago he had an accident in which he injured his back. This resulted in him being off work and then developing sleeping problems that have become chronic. He is now completely exhausted and very depressed.

Three different human beings. Three different insomnia scenarios but are there some patterns here?

Over the years, my experience has led me to come up with a model of insomnia that I call an Insomnia Spiral. This model enables me to roughly gauge the severity of my clients' sleep problems and then to come up with a possible treatment plan. It also helps me to assess how long it might take to sort the problem out.

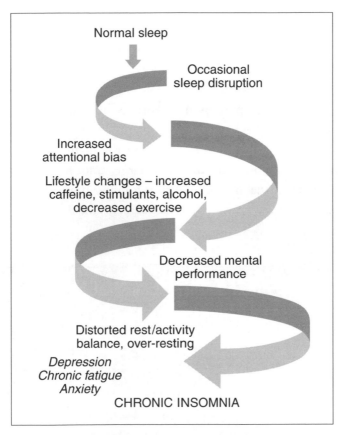

Figure 5: The Insomnia Spiral

In this model, we may all, from time to time, find ourselves surfing in and out between normal sleep and occasional sleep disruption. But what happens if the problems persist?

In the Insomnia Spiral certain events, lifestyle or behavioural changes can send an individual further into the spiral and return to normal sleep becomes more difficult. For example, a typical scenario might be that we are going through a stressful phase at work, we start experiencing the odd bad night of sleep, and occasional sleepiness becomes a more pervasive tiredness.

Insomnia worsens if the individual starts using alcohol or drugs to get to sleep and stimulants such as caffeine or energy drinks to stay awake and alert. Energy levels drop as sleep quality worsens and the individual becomes stuck in a 'fatigue' cycle (figure 6). A large part of my work is helping people with addictions who also have sleep problems and this fatigue cycle is often part of the picture. But for them, the pattern has become a lot more extreme with large amounts of alcohol, cocaine, marijuana and other drugs locking them deeper into the cycle.

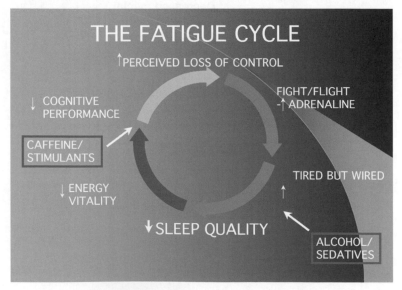

Figure 6: The Fatigue Cycle

Accompanying these events are the biochemical and physiological changes that occur as the internal chemistry essential for optimal sleep becomes disrupted. The sympathetic nervous system becomes over-active and the parasympathetic nervous system, which, as I have mentioned before, is vital for sleep, shuts down. As fatigue worsens, the individual finds it harder and harder to be active and increasingly spends time resting or, as I call it, over-resting. Over-resting reduces the body's need for actual sleep and the patient goes to bed, finds himself unable to sleep and the cycle worsens.

If you are reading this book because you are Tired but Wired, I'm sure you will be able to relate to at least some of this. Remember, many of us may experience occasional sleeplessness – we surf into the spiral and then bounce back out but those with chronic insomnia become stuck in the spiral and it becomes harder and harder to restore equilibrium particularly if other complications then arise such as physical or psychological problems and mood disorders (anxiety or depression). Some of my clients then end up on a cocktail of prescribed or even over-the-counter medications that not only affect their mood and morale but also their sleep.

STOP TRYING SO HARD!

A further complication in the development of insomnia arises when sleep begins to take too much of a centre stage. What I mean by this is that the person begins to develop anxiety about not sleeping and then starts making more of an effort – in fact, too much of an effort – to sleep. They might say, 'I slept so badly last night. I hope it doesn't happen again.' Or 'I must get to bed early and get some good sleep.' Of course the underlying worry is, 'Am I going to sleep tonight?!' Psychologists refer to this as *attentional bias,* meaning that the more we give something our attention the more significant it becomes. In the case of sleep, something that should happen so automatically and naturally, the more we become anxious about not sleeping the *less effort-less* it becomes.

Now there are some things we all need to make an effort to do in order to prepare ourselves for good sleep and I will remind you of some of these when we get to the Sleep Toolkit. But trying *too hard* can actually work against us getting good sleep. *Trying* to sleep is not sleeping and the more we try to sleep the more elusive sleep becomes. A crucial part of my work with my clients often involves helping them to let go and find the right level of effort needed to enable their sleep.

Previously I mentioned Paul the night shift worker whose insomnia started when he hurt his back. He is a classic case of 'trying too hard'. In fact, his problems with insomnia are some-what unusual in that he is actually spending enough time in bed and resting but is permanently exhausted. He has become quite obsessed with getting more sleep and he feels that he 'really needs' his sleep. His pre-sleep routine involves 'getting into bed by 9pm at the latest and watching at least one episode of his favourite comedy programme'. He becomes very anxious if there is any deviation from this routine and really believes that if he tries harder to sleep – gets to bed earlier or lies in for longer – he will start to feel better. One of the things I have been trying to do with him is break the cycle of fatigue by actually getting him to move *more* by taking more exercise, rest *less* and go to bed a little later – to actually take some of the emphasis off sleep.

I'm sure that you too have experienced a minor form of sleep-disrupting *attentional bias* yourself. Perhaps the night before a big presentation or exam when you tell yourself, 'I *must* get to bed early and get some good sleep tonight,' and then of course you spend the whole night tossing and turning and fretting about the sleep you so badly need!

Common Sleep Challenges

Here are some more common sleep challenges that my clients face. I wonder if you can relate to any of these.

NON-RESTORATIVE SLEEP

What most of us want and need is pure, refreshing 'clean' sleep. Sleep that is unmuddied by the information, noise, and worries of the day. Sleep that is unmuddied by chemical stimulants – caffeine, coca cola, 'energy' drinks, nicotine, alcohol and recreational drugs.

KEITH THE IT MANAGER

'Come on! I've got to have a life!' I heard this recently from a particularly exhausted client who visited my clinic for help with his sleep. 50-year-old Keith hadn't been sleeping well for years and was overweight and suffering from high blood pressure. He worked an intense 12-hour day with very few breaks, leaving the house at 7am and getting home at 7pm. After supper and 'a couple of gin and tonics' he passed out on his favourite chair in front of the TV, snored his way through his favourite crime programmes until he woke with a start around 2am and dragged himself up to bed. He then struggled to get to sleep until his alarm went off at 6am.

Unfortunately, my work with Keith was short-lived. He simply wasn't prepared to give up the cocktail of coffee and caffeinated energy drinks he lived on during the day, he wasn't prepared to acknowledge that he was probably drinking more than a couple of gin and tonics every evening and he certainly wasn't prepared to rethink his relationship with his BlackBerry which he kept switched on and under his pillow all night!

Clearly, Keith's sleep had become very muddied and this was

taking its toll not just on his energy levels but also on his health. I have no doubt that his weight and blood pressure problems were largely related to his lifestyle and sleep patterns. But he just couldn't and wouldn't change – the bad habits were too deeply ingrained.

Caffeine and Sleep

Caffeinated drinks have grown in popularity in the last decade and it is no coincidence that the coffee shop industry has grown exponentially as technology has taken off. Now don't get me wrong, I love a good cup of coffee and one of my favourite rituals is sitting in a café sipping at a nice cup of coffee while writing or watching the world go by. But for many of my clients, caffeine has become the biggest barrier to them getting good, clean sleep. I include in this tea, coffee, coca cola, caffeine tablets and caffeinated energy drinks even if they are masquerading as healthy 'vitamin shots'.

So what does caffeine do and how does it muddy your sleep? Caffeine acts very much like adrenaline so it revs up your sympathetic nervous system and increases the 'noise' of REM sleep – it disorders the memory consolidation process. Just imagine you've hired a hyperactive, wired, filing clerk for the day to sort your office out and imagine the chaos that might ensue and the mistakes he might make! Some of my clients have become so reliant on caffeine and they are getting sleep but it is noisy, buzzy disordered sleep that doesn't feel like sleep at all. The half-life of caffeine (the time taken for half of the caffeine to leave your body) is about 5hrs so you could have a cup of coffee at 5pm and still have half the caffeine in your system by 10pm. Now this might not be enough to make you the life and soul of the party but it might be enough to significantly affect the quality of your sleep.

Apart from the effect on your sleep, because of its adrenaline-like effect, caffeine also makes you more anxious and jittery. I've encountered far too many patients at the hospital who are being treated for anxiety disorders and panic attacks who are drinking huge amounts of caffeine. While undoubtedly they are facing some serious problems in their lives, the caffeine is not helping and in fact, it simply amplifies the anxiety and worry. When you get to the Sleep Toolkit, you will learn exactly how much caffeine is 'too much' and how to go about breaking a caffeine habit if you have one.

Alcohol and Sleep

For centuries, human beings have relied on alcohol as a relaxant and to ease our passage into sleep but if you suffer from sleep problems this might not be the best strategy. I don't want to be a complete killjoy and I enjoy a nice glass of wine as much as the next person but from a physiological perspective *any* alcohol will affect your sleep. The question is the degree to which it affects your sleep and can you get away with it? If you don't have any heavy demands on you the next day you may well get away with having less than optimal sleep. However, if you need to be firing on all cylinders you may need to think about your alcohol consumption. Personally, I *never* drink the night before I run workshops or face a packed schedule at the hospital. Having said that, I've had one glass too many the night before running a marathon, slept badly and still ran a great race the next day. It just goes to show, sleep is only one way of recovering energy!

Alcohol affects your sleep by affecting the brain chemicals or neurotransmitters needed for peaceful sleep. A nightcap of say one unit* may help to reduce the amount of time taken to fall

---

* 1 unit of alcohol is equivalent to a glass of wine, half a pint of beer or a single measure of spirits

asleep – the so-called *sleep latency*. However, even a trace presence of alcohol in the bloodstream can disrupt the second half of your sleep cycle, leading to wakefulness in the middle of the night and an inability to fall back to sleep. The important information consolidation process that takes place during REM sleep is also disrupted – imagine having a drunk filing clerk in your office! Such disturbances lead to daytime fatigue, which can affect your ability to undertake such everyday tasks as driving a car. Alcohol consumed *up to six hours before bedtime can still disturb one's sleep cycle that evening*. Unfortunately, the majority of alcohol consumption takes place from dinner on, leaving many susceptible to a fitful night.

The bottom line is that if you are suffering from persistent sleep problems, avoid alcohol until you have sorted them out. Some of my work involves working with alcoholics many of whom have problems with insomnia – they will have been using alcohol in order to fall asleep, but a reliance on alcohol leads to wakefulness later in the night, a compounded inability to fall back to sleep and a reliance on yet more alcohol to help them get back to sleep.

Finally, there's a connection between the sleep-related breathing disorder called *obstructive sleep apnea* and alcohol consumption. Drinkers can experience apnea if only for a night. Alcohol impairs breathing in sleep by relaxing the throat muscles and it affects the brain's breathing centre by masking the effect of low oxygen levels in the bloodstream, possibly damaging tissue. Even people who normally don't snore do so if they have been drinking the night before. Snorers without apnea can exhibit apnea symptoms if they have been drinking. Hangover symptoms – attributed to the efforts of the body to metabolise alcohol – are frequently partially due to breathing-disordered sleep.

I Can't Stop Moving!

'I get into bed exhausted and then I just can't stop moving! It feels almost as if something is crawling in my veins and it's absolutely maddening. The worse thing is that it stops me from falling asleep.'

Karen, 31 yr old mother of two young children.

Restless Legs Syndrome (RLS) is what can feel like strange sensations in your legs that stop you (and your bedmate) from sleeping. They may cause you to jump up and move around to relieve the discomfort. People who suffer from RLS complain of a creeping, crawling, tingling sensations in their legs. They also complain of feeling very tired throughout the day – their sleep simply isn't refreshing.

RLS syndrome is thought to be due to an imbalance in the nervous system – again the sympathetic nervous system becomes overactive and the parasympathetic becomes depressed and so sufferers will typically have problems resting, falling asleep and getting restorative sleep. Pregnant women may also suffer the symptoms of RLS. Estimates of how many people suffer from this syndrome range from 3-15%, with claims that it is under-reported and undiagnosed.

Similar to RLS is Periodic Limb Movement Disorder (PLMD) in which the sufferer experiences involuntary, rhythmic limb movements either while asleep or awake. While RLS disrupts sleep by delaying sleep, PLMD can disrupt sleep because of the constant limb movements. Often they don't even know that they are moving or twitching and it is their bed partner who notices it.

If you think you suffer from RLS or PLMD it may be worth a trip to your doctor to get to the root of the problem. You may even need a blood test as iron deficiency can cause some of the symptoms of RLS as can kidney disease. RLS can also be a side effect of some medications, including anti-depressants. A visit to a sleep laboratory may also help to determine whether you actually do suffer from RLS or PLMD and whether it is affecting your sleep.

While my work doesn't specifically involve diagnosing or treating these disorders I have noticed that they are more likely to occur under certain circumstances. For example, I have noticed that my clients who are very anxious, perfectionistic and somewhat controlling are more likely to suffer similar symptoms. These are often the individuals who are also working overtime at *trying* to sleep. Often one of the first traits I notice about them is their inability to just relax and let go. They find it hard to stop – either mentally or physically – and their lives are run by a mental list of 'must do's, should do's or have to do's'. Work with these individuals often involves helping them to stop, relax, breathe and let go and I have developed some specific exercises to help them which I will be sharing with you in my Sleep Toolkit.

When You Really Are Sleeping!

Earlier on I mentioned *paradoxical insomnia* – when you think you are not sleeping but you really are. I would like to tell you a little about this peculiar type of insomnia if only at least to offer you some reassurance that you may be getting more sleep than you think.

A while ago I was returning to the United Kingdom from a holiday in the Caribbean. I boarded the plane and reset my watch noticing that it was about 1.30am according to UK time which meant we had about seven and a half hours before we were due to touch down at the airport. I remember thinking to myself as I settled in, 'I really don't feel tired enough to sleep. I think I'm going to be watching a lot of films tonight.' The next thing I knew I awoke to the smell of coffee and the sound of the air stewardesses as they served breakfast! I had slept for over six hours.

When we sleep our perception of time becomes very skewed – a second can feel like an hour and an hour can feel like no time at all. This is what happens with paradoxical insomnia – your beliefs, expectations and worries about how much sleep you are or aren't getting actually get in the way of you getting sleep. At the hospital where I work, we have patients who are being checked regularly throughout the night by the night staff. The nurses tiptoe into the room to check that the patient is asleep and make a note in their records. The next morning the disgruntled and tired patient complains that they were awake all night! Often the patients feel angry and frustrated and demand to be given sleeping tablets the next night.

You may recall from the previous chapter that several times a night while we sleep we come into a shallow semi-conscious state called the hypnagogic trance and in this state we may feel as if we are fully awake when we are not.

I believe this is one of the most important phases of our sleep cycle and I pay special attention to this phase of sleep when working with sleep problems. For most of my clients, this mini-phase of sleep has become the 'enemy' – they get anxious, agitated and even panicky if they wake up. Often, they then adopt behaviours that keep them awake even longer such as checking the time, calculating (and worrying about) how many hours of sleep they will or won't get if they don't get back to sleep, and of course, checking the BlackBerry for messages.

Does this ring any bells for you? Of all of the bad sleep habits that I have encountered in my sleep practice, clock-watching is probably one of the habits most damaging to your sleep – and one of the hardest to break!

I recently worked with a 30yr old accountant who had been

experiencing problems with her sleep for over 5 years. She had no problems getting to sleep but would wake several times during the night and find herself unable to get back to sleep. At our first session she said, 'Last night I got two and a half hours of sleep. I was awake at 12, 3.30, and 4.45. I finally got to sleep at 5.30 this morning!'

I had a big task on my hands persuading this ardent clock-watcher to stop checking the time during the night. Even though she realised that her bad habits were getting in the way of her sleep she just couldn't stop doing it and she had two alarm clocks and her mobile phone to help her count the minutes away! 'I just need to know the time!' She would insist. By the time we got to our third session she had reluctantly agreed to relinquish the clocks and her sleep had already improved.

Hypersomnia or Over-sleeping

For some sleep problems can arise because they are actually 'over-sleeping'. It may be that they are getting to sleep too late and then sleeping late into the day which then starts to shift the whole circadian cycle – this is called *circadian rhythm sleep disorder* and is often seen with teenagers who are over-sleeping. I once had a 22yr old receptionist who came to see me complaining of 'needing more sleep' even though she was actually sleeping 12-13 hrs per night! I had to work hard to convince her to start cutting back on sleep, getting to bed earlier, waking up earlier and paying attention to other aspects of her energy such as nutrition and exercise.

Breathing Disorders

I place a great deal of significance on breathing patterns and techniques when I work with sleep and energy problems. Very early in my career in a physiology laboratory I noticed how so many factors can distort our breathing patterns and for some of my clients it is disrupted breathing that is causing some of their sleep problems. One of the more common ways in which this happens is with *snoring*. Others may have more severe breathing problems in which breathing is interrupted while sleeping and these 'breathing pauses' reduce the quality of sleep — this is called *sleep apnoea*. Typically sufferers will complain of feeling very sleepy during the day. Some of the factors I pay close attention to when treating such problems are abdominal weight, hydration levels (believe it or not, dehydration can cause snoring!) and, of course, breathing patterns.

Parasomnias – Nightmares, Night terrors and Teeth Grinding

Another group of sleep problems that I frequently encounter at my clinic is the *parasomnias*. These include teeth grinding or *bruxism*, nightmares and night terrors.

TEETH GRINDING

'The first time I heard it, I couldn't work out what it was,' said the wife of a business executive who had come to see me with sleep problems and fatigue, 'In the dark, it certainly did not sound human.'

The person who suffers from *bruxism* is often the last to know. The first to know is the spouse who shares the sufferer's bed — and is awakened by the rhythmic grinding of the teeth. The sufferer may visit his or her doctor with facial pain, ear-ache, neck pain or headache. But only a visit to the dentist will confirm the diagnosis, because the effects of bruxism are immediately visible on the teeth.

Bruxism is the unconscious nocturnal grinding of the teeth, but it is not just a dental problem. It can be a manifestation of deep-seated anxiety and tension. The dental implications can be promptly and effectively treated, and provided the sufferer sees a dentist soon enough, there should be no long-term effects. In severe cases, a gum-guard can be used. But the real treatment and cure lies in dealing with the root cause – the stress.

Often those who suffer from bruxism are perfectionist high-achievers who may have difficulties establishing and maintaining healthy boundaries in their work and home life – they simply find it difficult to say 'no'. Such individuals may also avoid asking for help and sharing their anxieties with others, even loved ones. They are the ones who sit quietly in my workshops, smiling serenely and letting everyone else give voice to their opinions.

Dentists will quickly spot the effects of nocturnal grinding. The jaw is an efficient crushing machine, and unconscious grinding can put thousands of pounds of pressure per square inch onto the teeth. Where enamel is destroyed, the dentin is exposed and the teeth can become sensitive. Teeth can be fractured. But grinding can be so severe that it threatens also the gum, underlying bone and jaw mechanism. Temporomandibular joint damage affects the hinge mechanism between the lower and upper jaw. This is why many bruxism sufferers have their symptoms in their jaws, ears and in the form of headaches.

The good news for those who manifest their stress as bruxism, is that it can be alleviated and prevented and the key to doing this is by learning how to express themselves. You will learn more about 'anti' bruxism techniques in the Sleep Toolkit but, in brief, when I work with children who have bruxism, the key to helping them often lies in getting them to express themselves creatively through art, singing, drama or even martial arts.

NIGHTMARES AND NIGHT TERRORS

With both nightmares and night terrors emotions are running high and the person may be quite distressed. The difference between the two lies in when it is that they occur; night terrors are likely to happen during deep sleep so the sufferer is often unaware of what is going on although they may appear to be fully awake and alert. Usually they can't remember what has happened afterwards but might be left with a bad feeling afterwards – an unpleasant aftertaste. Nightmares occur during REM sleep and because, as we learned in the previous chapter, this is a shallow stage of sleep, the individual is more likely to remember what they dreamt.

So is there help for those who are suffering from such things? Thankfully yes and my work with them often involves education, reassurance, and getting them to look at the lifestyle factors that will exacerbate the problem – such as caffeine and alcohol. Also, I often encourage my clients to 'make friends with their dreams and nightmares'. This may sound a little far-fetched but many of my clients are creative individuals who draw, paint, sing, or write. Some of them have creative talents that they haven't aired for decades. I encourage them to start paying attention to their creativity and invariably, the intensity of their dreams starts to abate. Perhaps, not surprisingly, one of the most popular treatments at the hospital is art therapy.

Un-Natural Sleep

Finally, a brief note about sleeping tablets . . .

Many of my patients at the hospital are on sleeping tablets and medication that will help them to sleep. Their sleep has become severely disrupted and they are in desperate need of some sleep. Taking sleeping tablets helps to 're-boot' the system but then many of them discover that after a while, the medication stops working and they might need an even higher dose to achieve the same sleep. In fact it is exactly for this reason that most medical practitioners advise taking medication for only two weeks – after this they tend to lose their efficacy. Apart from the loss of effectiveness, many patients also find that they experience unpleasant side effects – tiredness, nausea, dry mouth, dizziness, feeling like a 'zombie'. Some find that the tablets hardly work at all even at the outset.

Sometimes people come to see me and, understandably, they are desperate for solutions. They are desperate for me to give them something – a quick fix – that will give them the sleep that they crave. I recently met someone who was drinking a bottle of cough medicine *every night* to help him sleep. Being unable to sleep is horrible. There's nothing worse than lying in bed in the middle of the night, eyes hot and burning with fatigue, nausea gnawing at the pit of your stomach, worrying about how you are going to face the day ahead if you don't get some sleep.

The bottom line is that, although it might be necessary up to a point, taking sleep medication (or any other type of drug) *will never truly replicate your unique sleep system that is designed to give you the sleep that is exactly right for you.*

Just recently I was working with a group of patients in my clinic and a particularly tired-looking gentleman said to me:

'When I was sleeping well, I used to enjoy the feeling of just drifting off and then waking in the morning. It was such a delicious feeling and I want that back. But now that I am on sleeping tablets my sleep feels blunted somehow. I just fall asleep abruptly and then wake up – often tired and zombie-like. The tablets seem to be controlling my sleep almost mechanically.'

This made complete sense to me. Although this patient needed the sleeping tablets to aid his recovery, he knew that the sleep he was getting wasn't quite *his* sleep. Although at this time he may need the support of his medication, the time will come when we need to wean him off the sleeping tablets and to help his body and physiology to start producing his unique sleep again.

My aim is to guide you towards reconnecting with your unique sleep – the natural way. At the end of this book I have included some guidelines on weaning yourself off sleep medication – how to do it and what to expect. But please, I must emphasise that if you are thinking about stopping using any prescription drugs, you must consult your doctor before coming off them.

Sleep Overload

I hope you now have a good understanding of sleep problems and how they can arise. I want to end this section by returning to an issue you will recognise from earlier in the book.

This is to do with the burden we place on our sleep when we pay little or no attention to all of the other vital aspects of our energy and wellbeing. I refer to this as *sleep overload*. Sleep overload is created when:

1. We don't pay attention to other aspects of our health and energy and rely on sleep to do all the work of recovery;
2. We don't allow ourselves mental recovery time – there's no oscillation in our day.

Although sleep overload is not an established sleep disorder as such, it is a problem that I increasingly encounter in my clinic and that has convinced me that a powerful route to brilliant sleep is to pay attention to every aspect of our health – physical, mental, emotional and spiritual. After all, sleep *is* only one way in which we recover energy.

In the next chapter you will learn exactly how to renew and recover your energy on all of these levels. Trust me, this will not only improve your health and vitality but you will also discover the art of sleeping brilliantly.

REMEMBER:

- The most common forms of insomnia are difficulty getting to sleep, difficulty staying asleep and non-restorative sleep.
- Everyone experiences poor sleep from time to time.
- Good sleep is created by applying the right amount of effort. Trying too hard to sleep is actually disruptive.
- Caffeine and alcohol can stop you from getting deep, restorative sleep.
- Sleep problems can be caused by thinking we are not sleeping when in fact we are. This is called paradoxical insomnia.
- We can sleep brilliantly if we take the load off our sleep and pay attention to other aspects of our health and energy.

CHAPTER 4

Sleep is only one way of recovering energy!

In this chapter we are going to move away from sleep and take a look at all of the other ways in which you are able to renew your energy. Don't get me wrong, I believe that there is virtually nothing that can replace a good night's rest. However, your energy and the way you are feeling right now isn't just about how well you slept last night or even how you have been sleeping recently. It is far more complex than that and I hope that even though it may be your problems with sleep that have brought you to this book, you will take the time to read this section.

Learning about how to manage your energy could be the vital element that makes a big difference to your sleep.

Who needs a good night's sleep?

We are remarkably well-equipped to deal with poor sleep from time to time and as you learnt in the previous chapter, everyone has the odd bad night.

Now this might sound a little odd in the light of everything I've said about sleep and how important it is for your health and wellbeing. However, the spiral into insomnia can be caused by simply *trying too hard* to sleep. Often, an important part of my work is about helping my clients to see that they can actually cope with occasional bad sleep – particularly if they start to pay attention to other aspects of their energy. This means helping them to see that their sleep is only one (albeit vital) part of the picture and that they are far more resourceful than they might think . . .

What do I mean by 'resourceful'? I am sure you can relate to times when you haven't slept well but still felt fine the next day – maybe you even 'performed' at your best!

The following are just a few powerful examples of how well-equipped we are to cope with bad sleep:

- The professional footballer who scores the winning goal for his country despite a poor night's sleep in an unfamiliar hotel and country;
- The student who stays up all night to study and excels in her exams;
- The exhausted mother with a newborn baby surviving on very little sleep for the first year of her baby's life (I still remember this one!);
- Ellen MacArthur sailing the Vendee Globe solo in 2002, surviving on very little sleep and creating a new round the world record.

I'm sure that if you think hard about it you could probably find some of your own personal examples to add to this list.

Earlier on I shared with you some theories on how evolution has influenced our sleep and the need for resourcefulness if we couldn't sleep or rest. So what other energy resources do we have?

Perhaps I should begin by defining what I mean by 'energy'. In scientific terms, energy is defined most simply as the capacity to do work. I prefer to think of it as the *ability to live life to its fullest capacity.*

Carol – The Musician

A forty-year-old mother of two young children and musician, Carol had been referred by her doctor to see me for sleep problems that had been ongoing for three years. She had great difficulty getting to sleep and when she did her sleep was restless and fitful. She got out of bed most mornings feeling tearful, anxious and drained of energy and dreading going through the same cycle again at night. She was taking prescription sleeping tablets to help her sleep and was very anxious about giving them up. When I met Carol she came across as an attractive and gifted woman who had clearly lost her spark.

At our first session, I asked Carol to tell me about her lifestyle – she described a busy day organising the home and her family, very little rest during the day, snatched meals, no exercise (she once enjoyed jogging and playing tennis but had no energy now that she wasn't sleeping). Throughout the day she had a few cups of tea and coffee to keep her going. In the evening when her husband returned from his work in the City, she retired to her studio to work late writing and practising her music. On nights when she played gigs – perhaps a few times a month – she would get home at 2 or 3am exhausted but unable to sleep.

'I can't go on like this,' she said tearfully. 'I'm irritable with my husband and the kids. I don't even enjoy my music anymore!'

Clearly she was in a bad situation so we set to work immediately. The first thing I got Carol to think about was how she was *investing* in her energy. So leaving the issue of sleep (or rather, lack of it) to one side, what was she doing to fund all of the energy that her hectic life demanded? Carol realised that she hadn't been doing nearly enough and her 'homework' after our first session was to start taking small steps towards renewing her energy – she started getting out of bed a little earlier (albeit with some difficulty for the first week or so) to eat breakfast, she cut down on her cups of tea and coffee, she started drinking more water, snacking healthily during the day especially if she was going to be working late and taking a little time out – even if just 10 mins – to sit down and eat some lunch.

And the outcome? At our second session two weeks later Carol looked like a different woman – her spark had returned. 'The sleep's still a problem but I feel so much better!' she said. 'I've even played tennis and gone running a few times *and* I seem to have fallen in love with my family again!' At this point I knew that Carol was ready to start working with me on her sleep – she had stabilised her energy levels, taken the pressure off her sleep and we were now ready to start using some power tools to get her sleeping well.

A little while ago I received an email from Carol:

'I'm now off the sleeping tablets and sleeping well most nights. If I do get a bad night now and then, I don't let it phase me and my energy is still good the next day. Often I just use the time to rest and relax and think about my music and then, of course, I just end up falling asleep!'

You and your energy

I hope that Carol's story has started to get you thinking about you and your energy levels . . .

Over the years, I've been lucky enough to work with thousands of different types of people – some of them have an abundance of energy and resilience and just seem to cope incredibly well with the challenges life throws at them. On the other hand, some of them get burnt out, chronically fatigued and stressed. A lot of people fall somewhere between these extremes.

WHERE WOULD YOU PUT YOURSELF ON THIS 'ENERGY SCALE'?

I've always been fascinated by the habits of this 'high energy' group. What are they getting right (because I want to join this group myself)? Is there something that this 'low energy' group is getting wrong?

When I first began looking for answers to these questions, it became clear that although sleep played a big part in the energy story, it wasn't just about sleep. It became clear that *sleep is only one way of getting energy.* Those who occupied the high energy group seemed to have a wide range of energy-harnessing habits while those in the low-energy group seemed to rely heavily on getting sleep to give them their energy. I also discovered that by getting this latter group to rethink their views on sleep and look at the other ways in which they were renewing their energy they could actually end up getting better sleep – just as Carol did!

Right now I want you to think a little bit more about your energy . . .

What are your energy levels like *right now*?

On a scale of 1 to 10 (1 being the 'low energy group' and 10 being the 'high energy group'), what score would you give yourself right now?

My next (and most important question) is what have you

done to invest in your energy today? How have you created the score you have? If it is above 7 what are you getting right? If it is below 5 what could you do to give yourself more energy?

These are questions I ask my clients when they complain of feeling tired and burnt out. Sometimes they tell me about the breakfast they had (or didn't have), how many cups of coffee they've drunk, how they slept last night, and so on. Naturally, what we eat and drink can have a significant impact on how we feel but there are so many other ways in which we can nourish or drain our energy.

The Energy Pyramid

Over the years I've used an **Energy Pyramid** to provide a framework for the energy solutions that I recommend to my clients. I've borrowed and adapted this model from psychologist Abraham Maslow's 'Hierarchy of Needs'. Maslow, the grandfather of social psychology, asked the question, 'What do human beings need?' He identified needs which sit at different levels of a pyramid – at the bottom of the pyramid are the basic, physical needs such as food and warmth and at the top are the greatest needs such as our spiritual needs.

I've found that this pyramid offers a useful way of identifying what we need to stop ourselves from burning out. It will also help you to identify clearly where the gaps are and to think more creatively and holistically about how you can care for yourself better.

Here is a brief summary of how the pyramid works and while you read this I want you to think about the energy 'levels' and how they relate to you:

The Energy Pyramid

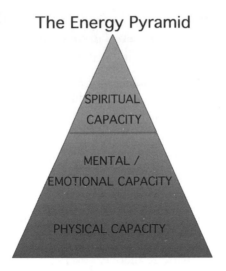

Figure 7: The Energy Pyramid

The Physical capacity energy level – this is the base level
of the pyramid and represents the foundations of **your**
energy. It is related to how we sleep, our fitness levels,
nutrition, rest and recovery. In other words, the basic
things we do to care for ourselves physically and the things
that give us our vitality and make us feel physically well
and energised.

Emotional capacity – This level is related to your emotional
health and energy – self-awareness and your ability to
manage negative emotions such as guilt, worry, fear and
anger. It is related to how you nourish positive energy-
enhancing emotions such as joy, happiness, and love and
build healthy and supportive relationships, particularly
with those who are nearest and dearest to you.

Mental capacity – This next level is related to the ways in
which we think and problem solve, nourish ourselves
intellectually, and manage our relationship with control and

perfectionism. It is related to how we deal with uncertainty and generate optimism even in times of adversity.

Spiritual capacity – This sits at the top of the pyramid and is the highest source of your energy. I'm often asked 'what is spiritual energy?' and it can be difficult to describe because it is so deeply personal to each and everyone. Some say it is when you feel at peace with life, a sense of joy and happiness deep within, feeling contented and centred in yourself. This is the energy that is unleashed when you tap into your deepest values, when you are doing what you truly believe in. It is the energy that sustains us throughout adversity and is our greatest source of motivation, determination and resilience.

I've been working with this 'pyramid' model for many years now and it offers me a powerful way of working not just with my clients' energy levels but also with their sleep problems – sleep problems can be caused by imbalances at any of the levels of the pyramid. Let me illustrate this by telling you about Helen's sleep problems and how we set about using the principles of the Energy Pyramid to put them right.

Helen's Sleep Problems

A few years ago Helen, a 31 yr old lawyer, came to see me about her sleep problems that had developed since qualifying as a solicitor 3 years ago. She looked and felt exhausted. Worst of all, she was thinking of abandoning the successful career which she had once enjoyed because of her anxiety that her fatigue would get in the way of her being able to work or cause her to make critical mistakes. She had been to her doctor who had given her sleeping tablets that a) she wasn't happy about taking and b) didn't seem to be working anymore.

When Helen met me she was desperate for help and as soon as she entered the consulting room she started pouring out her problems.

Helen's difficulties started as soon as she got into bed when her brain just seemed to come alive and she just couldn't fall asleep even though she was exhausted (a classic case of Tired but Wired). Eventually she would fall asleep but wake constantly throughout the night, each time finding it more difficult to get back to sleep and worrying about her ability to face work the next day. Finally, she would fall into a deep sleep around 5.30 in the morning and getting out of her bed when her alarm went off at 6.45 was impossible. After pressing her snooze button at least five times, Helen would jump out of bed in a panic, skip breakfast and leave for work feeling tired, and not particularly looking forward to the day ahead.

She would arrive at work at about 9am and, fuelled by the coffee and muffin she picked up along the way, she was ready to face the day. Lunch was inevitably a snatched sandwich at her desk, biscuits left over from meetings or completely forgotten. Coffee and chocolate would get her through the rest of the day and she rarely got home before 9pm. Work increasingly had been crowding into her weekend and this had worsened since she was given a BlackBerry, as she was then constantly accessible.

(In fact, at our first session it took some persuading to get Helen to relinquish her grip on her BlackBerry. She eventually agreed to put it on silent mode and place it on the table where she could glance at it from time to time.)

Helen would spend her evenings slumped in front of the TV with a glass or two of wine and a takeaway. In the past she would go to the gym a few times a week. Of late, she would fall asleep on the sofa and then drag herself to bed where she would toss and turn, unable to fall asleep.

We solved Helen's sleep problems by working at each of the levels of the pyramid.

At the **physical level**: There was a lot of work to be done here. I got Helen to take a hard look at what she was eating and drinking throughout the day. By cutting back on her caffeine and sugar intake and replacing them with healthy convenient snacks and low fat meals she noticed a positive shift in her energy levels. She also began eating breakfast first thing in the morning and drinking 1.5 litres of water per day. Once her energy had lifted, she was able to return to the gym and started doing some gentle yoga and relaxation exercises at home to prepare her for sleep.

At the **emotional level**: Helen started keeping a journal in which she could simply dump the worries and anxieties of the day. She found this especially helpful because she had become so isolated from her friends and family and she really found it difficult to talk to them about the problems she was experiencing at work.

At the **mental level**: Helen really needed to do some work on her time management and boundaries. She started to take small steps towards introducing some healthy habits into her working day – lunch breaks away from her desk, breaks during the day, not *always* working on the train, and definitely not going to bed with her BlackBerry beside her! She also started keeping a to-do list that she updated at the end of the day. This simply stopped her waking up during the night and worrying about the things she had to do the next day.

At the **spiritual level**: Although Helen wasn't having any major spiritual crises, and she actually enjoyed her job, she felt a little lost and life definitely held very little fun or excitement for her. She had lost touch with her friends and family and her one big passion in life, painting, had all but disappeared. Again, we looked at the small steps Helen could take towards rebuiliding her relationships and finding some time, however little, to return to her hobby.

I saw Helen again two months after we had had our last session. She was glowing with vitality, sleeping like a dream and living life to its fullest.

I hope you have found this a useful 'detour' from the subject of sleep and that you have taken some reassurance from understanding exactly how resourceful you are. I hope you are also starting to see that the problems you have been experiencing with your sleep may not be *exclusively* related to sleep and that paying attention to other aspects of your energy and lifestyle may actually take you closer to your goal of getting wonderful sleep.

REMEMBER:
- Sleep is only one way of getting energy;
- Your energy is nourished at several levels physical, mental, emotional and spiritual;
- Your sleep problems can be caused by imbalances at one or more of these levels;
- You can improve your sleep by addressing the imbalances at these levels;
- You can create brilliant health, energy and wellness by addressing the imbalances at these levels.

CHAPTER 5

Are You Ready To Take Control of Your Sleep?

We are what we repeatedly do.

- Aristotle

The fact that you have taken the time and effort to get hold of this book, read it and spend time getting to this page means that, on some level, you are ready to do the work on your sleep. *You are taking responsibility for your sleep.*

For many years I have been using my own mini-model to assess my clients' readiness for change. I call this the *ARC of Change* in which we first of all become **A**ware of our role in creating whatever situation we are in, we then take **R**esponsibility for changing our situation by making different **C**hoices. By making different choices, we create a different outcome. Are you ready to create your ARC of change?

```
Awareness

Responsibility

Choices
```

The ARC of Change

Before you open up the Toolkit, please take a moment to consider whether you really are ready to do the work on your sleep. Sometimes my clients are surprised when I ask this question – of course they want to start sleeping better but often, it is only when we start working together that they realize that they are going to have to start making some different choices. This may involve letting go of habits that you have become quite attached to and replacing them with habits that will help you to create the brilliant sleep that you deserve.

The following are just a few of the things my clients have told me over the years that convince me that they are NOT ready to do the work:

'I can't possibly switch my phone off at night! I have to check my messages.' I heard this from a 23yr old trainee solicitor who had been signed off from work with stress and burnout.

'But I need to know the time!' Unfortunately, still the most popular 'bad habit' that I regularly encounter (you will soon learn more about the hazards of nocturnal clockwatching).

'I'm not ready to give up my coffee/alcohol/drugs/partying etc. I've got to enjoy life after all!' Or *'I can't face breakfast in the morning – I've never been a 'breakfast eater.' In fact, no one in our family has ever been able to stomach breakfast in the mornings – it's in our genes!'*

Again, both popular comments. Now I'm not necessarily asking you to give up the things that you enjoy but just to reassess their role in your life and whether you really do need them.

I would also invite you to think about how much you really want brilliant sleep. In fact, what does 'brilliant sleep' mean for you? It is important to have a clear goal of what you want so that when you get to the Toolkit you can choose your sleep tools with this goal clearly in mind. It is also important to have a clear vision to help keep you on track and stop you lapsing back into unhelpful, sleep-disrupting patterns of behaviour.

Hold the vision

If we have a vision for where we want to go, then our behaviour is more likely to follow that direction. I call this the 'power of intention'. It's a bit like playing golf – you look to the spot where you want to hit the ball (create the vision) and then swing through to hit that spot.

So what is your intention for your sleep? What would be your vision of wonderful, deeply restorative sleep? This may sound like an odd thing to have to think about but you may find that you already have an unconscious vision but *it might be one that isn't actually helpful for your sleep.* For example,

> *'I don't want to wake during the night,' or 'I hope my neighbours don't wake me up again,' or 'I'm so worried that I won't sleep tonight and I've got such a big day tomorrow.'*

In each of these cases, the vision of *not* getting bad sleep creates exactly that – bad sleep! This is because you become so focused on what you *don't* want. Rather like saying 'Don't think of pink elephants!' And I'll bet that right now you can't get the image of marauding pink elephants out of your head!

So back to the important question: What does 'brilliant sleep' mean for you?

To help you answer this question allow me to offer you my version of what I think it means . . .

For me, brilliant sleep means putting my head on the pillow, sliding effortlessly into thick, velvety, comforting sleep, occasionally waking up, briefly enjoying the sensation of being cosy and comfortable before returning to my cocoon of sleep, and then, finally waking up feeling rested and revitalised and looking forward to the day ahead — regardless of the number of hours of sleep I have had.

Doesn't that sound wonderful? Start thinking about it now. You might like to use a journal or notepad to start creating your vision of brilliant sleep. Feel free to modify it as you read on and learn more about your sleep but for now, just go for it. The sky is the limit!

I would also encourage you to keep this somewhere that you can look at it often. One of my clients, a sleep-deprived mother of three young children, would write her sleep vision words on bits of sticky paper and then place them all over the house to remind her of exactly what she was working towards. This reminded her that she needed to slow down, breathe and relax even while on the go.

In case you are struggling a little with being able to create your vision, here are a few words to help you along the way. Feel free to make them your own:

Soft	Thick	Refreshing
Peaceful	Nourishing	Blissful
Comforting	Smooth	Deep
Velvety	Rich	Soothing

Don't forget, I also want to help you to have more energy and vitality. So your vision for your sleep might also reflect this. As one of my clients recently, and memorably, said to me: 'I want to have the kind of sleep that gives me the energy to live every bit of my life to the full. I want to wake up each morning looking forward to the day ahead!' This client actually made a beautiful collage of his favourite things in life – his family, mountain biking, his garden, the sea – to remind him of what he wanted to enjoy in life and what better sleep could bring him. This helped him to keep on track whenever he felt himself lapsing back into bad habits.

Assessing Your Level of Motivation

How ready are you to make the changes necessary to create your brilliant sleep? How motivated are you?

There are several stages in the process of change. Take a look at the flow diagram in Figure 8 and try to gauge exactly where you are in this model. I always ask my clients to consider where they might be in this change model. Occasionally, upon reflection, they realise that they just aren't ready to do the work and I never see them again.

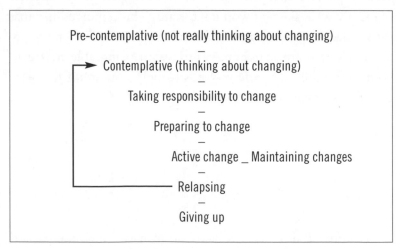

Figure 8: Assessing your motivation to change

'My life is just a bit too hectic at the moment. I'll come back to see you when things get a bit quieter.' I heard this from a 34-year-old optician who ran his own busy practice. The problem was he was the sort of person who was always going to be busy. The other problem was he had been taking sleeping tablets on and off for over 5 years – he knew it wasn't a good idea and that they weren't helping him to sleep anyway.

'I'm quite happy with my sleep, thank you very much!' This came from Keith the IT manager I mentioned earlier. Keith had been coerced into coming to see me by his family who were fed up of seeing him regularly downing his nightly gin and tonics, passing out on the sofa and then struggling to sleep when he did get into bed at 2am. Keith wasn't even considering making any changes to his sleep habits and wasn't going to waste his or my time by coming to see me again.

Can you see where you are on this change model? To help you to work this out, the following are just some of the things you might say to yourself depending on your level of commitment:

Pre-contemplative	I've got this condition so there's nothing I can do about it. It's in my genes/ it runs in the family.
Contemplative	Can I really do this? What do I stand to gain by making these changes? What will I lose?
Taking responsibility	What do I need to do?
Preparing to change	How am I going to go about this? What support do I need? What day will I start?
Active change/ Maintaining change	What changes am I noticing? Am I getting closer to my vision? Am I making progress?

Relapsing	Is this really going to make a difference anyway?
	Is this really worth it?
Giving up	What's the point anyway?

You have to make it imperative

What do I stand to gain by changing my current patterns of
  behaviour?
What do I stand to lose?
What could better sleep and/or more energy bring to my
  life?

Can you link your goals to something that for you holds a
deeper purpose or meaning? What would better sleep mean for
you? More energy to do the things you enjoy doing? More
energy for the people you care about? Write it down or even
make a poster. Make sure you look at it several times a day to
remind yourself of your intention.

What to expect

An important part of my work with my clients involves man-
aging their expectations of what will happen once they start
doing their sleep work. This is often key to helping them to
avoid relapsing back into their old unhelpful habits.

So what should you expect?

Some of my clients notice immediate improvements in their
sleep when they start using the sleep tools. For others, the
process is slow and it can feel as if you are taking two steps forward and one step back.

If your sleep has been getting worse over a long period of
time it can take a little while to get it back on course – it may

not happen (literally) overnight. But it can be done! Keep holding on to your vision and don't give up hope. Just as your sleep is unique to you, when you begin to repair your sleep each one of you can expect something different to happen. Here are just a few of the things you can expect:

1. **Nothing happens** – or at least, it may feel as if nothing is happening. You might feel like giving up or reverting to taking your sleeping tablets (or anything else you might have been using) to help you sleep. The important thing is to persevere, keep using the tools and don't give up.

2. **Nothing happens to your sleep but you feel better** – this is a result that I often see if my patients have been stuck in the fatigue cycle I described earlier. Many of the changes you will make affect other aspects of your energy – emotional, mental or spiritual. It is not unusual for me to hear my client say after a few days of using the sleep tools: 'My sleep is still not brilliant but it doesn't seem to bother me as much.' Or, 'I didn't sleep well last night but I feel fine today and I seem to have lots of energy.' This response is quite common and often it comes with a *softening of attitude* towards sleep that tells me we are heading in the right direction. This positive shift is often the vital stage that precedes sleep improvement.

3. **One brilliant night of sleep!** And then you revert back to your original disrupted pattern of sleep. Occasionally this happens *straight after* my patients start using the tools. Why this happens I'm not sure – one of my theories about this is that the brain is offering up a bit of encouragement for you and helping you to create a vision of what your brilliant sleep can feel like.

4. **Some improvement** – For example, you might find that you are able to fall asleep easily but still wake in the night

and find it hard to get back to sleep. When you get to the Toolkit you will see that there are different 'grades' of tools – ones that are easy to use and ones that take a bit more time and effort to get the hang of. Often it is these latter tools that will help to get the more persistent problems sorted. The key is to keep on track and keep working on it.

5. **Brilliant sleep returns!** Naturally it would be fantastic if all of my clients could experience this result but the reality is that it doesn't always work this way. For some of my more fortunate clients good sleep returns almost immediately – often these are individuals who have once slept well (they might even have been Martini sleepers) who experienced some stress or trauma which upset the balance of their sleep. In the process, they might also have developed some bad habits that exacerbated the problem. For them, brilliant sleep returns speedily and it is rare for me to see these clients after two sessions.

People respond in different ways once they start using the Sleep Toolkit. Sometimes even I am not clear why I get the results I do but it does reinforce my belief that there is still so much to learn about the mysterious and wonderful process of sleep.

And finally, just a few thoughts to keep you on the right path . . .

Resetting the pilot light

A while ago, the boiler in our heating system at home started malfunctioning – sometimes it worked perfectly, at other times, for no particular reason, it stopped working. There seemed to be no rhyme nor reason to its playing up. We called in a service engineer who poked and prodded around in the heating cupboard, tutted a few times and then said the dreaded words 'This might need replacing.' Of course, this isn't what we wanted to hear at all – replacing a boiler is expensive business! After some thought he said 'Let's try replacing this part and see if it does the trick.' So he did this and for the next 48 hours the boiler groaned and protested as it tried to get used to the change. It produced the heating and hot water but it certainly complained about it. Eventually it settled down and, so far, has been running like a dream.

I often use this analogy of my boiler system with my clients when I am trying to help them understand what is happening when we get to work on their sleep. It can be like restoring a vital connection in your 'sleep circuit board' and it may not happen overnight. Your sleep might feel 'cranky' or unpredictable. It might groan and creak as you begin to restore your sleep.

Treat your sleep like the British weather!

I have used this expression before but there's no harm in repeating it – if you can hold this thought at the back of your mind while you use the sleep tools you stand a better chance of being successful with your sleep.

At the time of writing Tired but Wired and against all predictions, Britain has been experiencing unusually heavy snowfall – in fact the heaviest for two decades according to Met records.

It is important that you manage your expectations of what will happen once you start using the sleep tools. Some nights you will sleep well, some nights your sleep will be neither good nor bad, other nights, against all predictions (i.e. you've done all the right things) it might be awful. And that's just the way it is. A bit like the British weather.

Knowledge is not wisdom

Information is not knowledge. Knowledge is not wisdom.
                                                        – Frank Zappa

I love this saying and it so beautifully sums up one of the things that can so often get in the way of getting great sleep. I have worked with sleep-deprived individuals who are so knowledgeable on the subject of sleep that they have taught me a thing or two! I once worked with a lovely lady who was a retired nurse. She had terrible problems with her sleep and she was a walking encyclopedia on the subject of sleep disorders. '*My problem is that I know all of this stuff but I just don't do it*'. Your problems with sleeping may have led you to read and learn a great deal about the subject but don't forget – you've got to put it into practice. And practice, practice, practice to take you closer to your vision of brilliant sleep.

Small changes, big results

Before you move on to start work with the Toolkit, I would like to offer you a few words of encouragement and this is that small changes really can make a big difference. I have seen this countless times with my clients – their sleep improves immeasurably and they are not even sure why because the changes they have made are so small as to seem almost insignificant. If you are tired, overwhelmed and not really sure where to start I hope you can take heart from this. Don't be put off by what might seem like an insurmountable task – small changes really can make a big difference.

REMEMBER:

- Your motivation is key to your success
- Don't give up, create and hold a strong vision of what your brilliant sleep could be like. Keep coming back to your vision if you feel your motivation slipping
- Be prepared and manage your expectations – sleep can be unpredictable – like the British Weather
- Small changes really can make a big difference

Part Two

THE SLEEP TOOLKIT

You should now have a greater understanding of your sleep and be starting to gather some insight into how you can improve as well as develop a healthier relationship with it.

This section is dedicated to the Sleep Toolkit.

The techniques come from a *holistic* toolkit that I have been developing and using with thousands of clients over the years. I also use them to give me the good sleep, energy and resilience to write this book and meet all of the other commitments in my busy life.

Some of the tools may be familiar to you but by organising them into this toolkit, I'm hoping to make it easier for you to select the ones that, over time, will be absolutely right for you. This is not a 'one size fits all' approach: I'm going to show you how to select those that are just right for you based on the knowledge you have learnt about your sleep. In this way, you will start to put together your own **unique sleep toolkit**.

Working with so many sleep problems has enabled me to 'group' the sleep tools into different 'compartments' according to how easy they are to use, the kind of results they will produce, and the sorts of problem they can be used to treat. Each of these has been tested by my clients and myself, and complementing each section I will also share with you their personal stories of the successful application of the tools.

Toolkit Contents

The **Nuts and Bolts Tools** include the essential habits and routines that we all need to be practicing in order to sleep well; they lay the foundations for your sleep. Much of what you will learn here is about creating the optimal *external environment* for your sleep. I would recommend that you first take a look in here. Are you already using these tools? If not, then this is where the work must begin for you. Please don't be tempted to skip this section – some of the tools in this 'compartment' may seem minor but they might provide the one element that can really make a big difference to your sleep.

I consider the **Basic Tools** to be the equivalent of the hammer or screwdriver in a builder's toolkit as these are the tools that I hope you will be using most of the time to help you to sleep well. **The Power Tools** are the equivalent of the builder's electric drills and will help to refine and optimise the quality of your sleep taking it to the next level.

The Basic and Power Tools work by helping you to create the optimal *internal environment* for your sleep. You have learnt that your internal chemistry needs to be just right in order for you to get good sleep. This is the precise cocktail of hormones, bio-chemical messengers and nerve pathways that is *unique* to you only. You can restore this internal chemistry by using the tools in this toolkit.

Toolkit Instructions

Here are some brief instructions and then it's over to you to start selecting your tools and putting them to use:

- Take time to examine each tool – no matter how small it may seem – and ask yourself if it might work for you. *Small changes really can make a difference.*
- Practice practice practice. The more you practice, the better results you will get.
- Don't be tempted to give up if you don't initially get results.
- Don't be tempted to give up if you *do* get the results you want. Keep using the tools until they become 'hardwired' into your behaviour. Until they become second nature. On average, it takes about **21 days** to create a habit. Try to practice each technique for at least 21 days unless otherwise specified.
- Make it imperative. Hold on to your vision of brilliant sleep.
- Try to use your natural intelligence – your inner voice – to work out what is right for you.

CHAPTER 6

The Nuts and Bolts

These are the tools that are absolutely essential for laying the foundations of your sleep. As I have said before while these rules may work for most people I want you to think about whether they really work for you. Tune in to that inner voice and ask yourself:

Would this make me feel comfortable and comforted?
Safe and secure?

Some of this may seem obvious, or you may be already doing some of these things without actually realising why. I hope this section will give you a greater understanding of why it is that there are some things you feel you *have* to do before you go to bed and, importantly, the role they play in creating your brilliant sleep.

Nuts and Bolts 1: Your wind down routine – entering the transition zone

The beginning holds the seed of all that is to follow.

– I Ching

Preparing to sleep is all about 'state preparation'. Just as an athlete warms their muscles up, stretches, focuses their mind, we need to prepare our minds and bodies in order to be able to sleep. The period before you go to bed – maybe the hour or two before – is what I often call the 'transition zone' as it creates a transition between the busyness of the day and the peace and stillness of night. A transition is a conscious pause. It is time to take stock of yourself and your day before moving into the next phase of rest. For many, this stillness becomes elusive if there is no transition, nothing to punctuate the end of the day's activity and the start of the period of rest and sleep. And how do we create this transition? By slowing down, by easing off the accelerator both physically and mentally.

I'm sure that you are familiar with the term 'winding down'. We should all have our own wind down practices – the rituals and routines that we go through before we go to bed that send an essential message to the brain *'It's time to let go of the day'* and, more importantly, *'It's safe to sleep.'* Sometimes my clients think they have no wind down routine and then I ask them if they do any of the following:

Check the front door is locked
Have a milky drink
Get your clothes ready for the next day
Switch your computer off
Tuck your children in bed and give them a final
    goodnight kiss

Clean your teeth
Pray

I then see the looks of recognition. We *all* have our favourite habits and routines, the things that we do to sign off the day – or at least we should do. Human beings are very ritualistic – not unlike our pets that have their preferred time to sleep, favourite corner, basket or rug and toys. It is these rituals and behaviours that create the feelings of safety that are the vital precursor to sleep.

Unhelpful Routines

I recently received an email from a 25yr old engineer who was desperate for some help with his sleep:

> 'I finish work at 10pm and then get home and eat (I know my diet is very poor), I then struggle to relax and sleep – I just can't switch my mind off. I eventually have to jump on the Internet, play Playstation or listen to some music. That process can take a few hours. Sometimes I get so anxious that I just get in the car and go out for a long drive. This means I don't get to sleep until 3 or 4am and I'm exhausted. Please help!'

Some of my clients have pre-sleep rituals but they are *unhelpful* and actually act as a barrier to getting good sleep. Do any of these sound familiar?

Negative Wind Down Rituals

- Working late then trying to get to sleep without allowing yourself some time to wind down.

- Working in bed on your laptop. I once had a client who really did this and not surprisingly, she was also experiencing some relationship problems.
- Having devices like mobile phones switched on and next to you in bed (or even under your pillow!).
- Watching TV in bed to put you to sleep. The frequency of TV waves is such that it is more likely to set your sleep pattern into a restless, shallow, 'thinking' type mode of sleep.
- Watching the 'wrong' type of TV before you get to bed – programmes that are violent, over-stimulating. Remember, the aim is to create a feeling of 'safety' before you go to bed.
- Reading the wrong books before you go to bed, the same principle as the wrong TV.
- Uncompleted business – getting up in the middle of the night to send emails, voicemails or write lists.
- Eating a heavy meal too soon before bedtime.
- Going to bed hungry.
- Strenuous, competitive exercise too soon before bedtime.
- Over-stimulating conversations in bed before you sleep.
- Going to bed with anger, bitterness and the worries of the day.
- Drinking large amounts of alcohol to help you get to sleep.
- Taking drugs (legal or otherwise) to help you get to sleep.

Helpful Routines

Now start thinking about your own rituals for winding down. The key question to ask yourself is: *What do I need to do in order to make me feel relaxed, calm and safe before I go to bed?*

To help you create your ideal wind down routine you might like to select some habits from the following list:

Positive Wind Down Rituals

Have a milky caffeine-free drink

Lay the breakfast table (your grandparents probably did this years ago)

Prepare your work clothes and pack your briefcase for the next day

Write a to-do list for the next day

Watch something on TV that is light and enjoyable but not too involving and over-stimulating but **switch the TV off at least half an hour before going to bed**

Read something that is light, philosophical, spiritual, life-affirming

Listen to music that is soothing and relaxing

Light a candle and meditate or pray

Nuts and Bolts 2: Your ideal sleep environment – preparing your 'cave'

Another essential nuts and bolts tool for good sleep is paying attention to your sleep environment. The important question for the 21st Century hunter-gatherer is 'how can I make my cave feel safe to sleep in?' This means making your physical space *just right* for you. When I was a student, I never knew why I could never 'sleep on the floor' when I went to parties. Whatever the time and regardless of my state of inebriation, like a homing pigeon, I had to make my way home. Now I understand that, as a Sensitive sleeper, it was essential for me to be in my own space and sleep environment unlike most of my friends (who were probably Martini sleepers anyway!).

So if you need to include the 'environment' tool in your sleep toolkit you need to pay attention to:

The lighting – make sure that it is just right for you. Do you need complete dark or do you like to wake up to some light (as I do).

The smell – using aromatherapy oils can help create a comforting, soothing, sleep-inducing space. When I am particularly busy I put a few drops of eucalyptus and lavender oils into a cup of hot water and place this in my bedroom about 20 minutes before I get into bed and the smell diffuses into the room.

The sound – you may awaken at the slightest noise if you are a sensitive sleeper in which case you might find it helpful to use some 'white noise' to block out external noises. White noise tracks can be downloaded from the internet (see Useful Resources) and often consist of natural sounds such as waterfalls, waves or the wind rustling in the trees. For some, another effective sound–minimiser is ear plugs. For many years I've slept with a fan on at night and, for me, this is the best form of white noise. Even during winter when it is colder I might just turn the fan towards the wall. The sound lulls me to sleep but most importantly, it stops me waking up at the slightest noise. I find this particularly helpful when I stay in unfamiliar environments such as hotels and often I will check with the hotel in advance and ask them to have a fan placed in my room.

Clutter – close your eyes and imagine your room right now. Is it a haven of peace and tranquillity or a jungle of chaos and unfinished business? If the latter, this may be contributing to your Tired but Wired sleep. Some people sleep blissfully in chaotic environments – teenagers' bedrooms often bear witness to this! But most of us need order and calm and as few reminders of the next day's work as possible. Many of my clients are writers and journalists and often I have to persuade them to try to separate their work from their sleeping space and I would invite you to do the same. If due to lack of space you do have to work in your bedroom, then can you try to create some boundaries between your work and rest? One journalist that I have worked with recently now places a white sheet over her desk and laptop when she has finished working. She also avoids working in her pyjamas and gets changed and starts winding down when the white sheet is in place.

Shared caves – now I have to mention the issue of sharing your bed because I get so many clients asking me whether it is best to sleep alone or share your bed with your partner. Sometimes my clients feel guilty about admitting that they actually sleep *better* on their own! We all have our preferred sleeping positions and sides of the bed. In fact, sleeping positions are deeply ingrained – the most common being the foetal position – and once established are rarely changed. Along with these preferences are the choices that we prefer to make about room temperature, lighting, and duvet thickness. It's a small wonder that any of us can get any sleep at all if we're sharing our bed!

My stance on this is that you should go with what is best for both of you (and most convenient). Many people actually sleep best on their own, undisturbed by the nocturnal noises and movements of their bedmates. For some of my more exhausted patients, I even recommend that they negotiate sleeping separately from their partners until they have normalised their sleep patterns and recovered some energy. On the other hand, I also have clients who have lost a partner through bereavement or separation and have subsequently developed sleep problems – for them, safety was linked to sharing their sleeping space with their partner. Their work is about building an inner core of safety in the absence of their loved one. You will learn about how to do this when you get to the Power Tools section of the Sleep Toolkit.

Temperature and air quality – ideally, in order for us to sleep well, there needs to be a fractional temperature difference between our body and our brain – a warm body and a cool head. Again, some of this boils down to personal preference and you may need to experiment with open windows, thickness of your duvet, choice of bedclothes, a fan on, air conditioning or your heating on or off or even how much clothing you wear. *Whatever you do the key is to keep warm in a cool room.*

Nuts and Bolts 3: Timing

What time are you naturally inclined to get into bed? Earlier I described to you the Owls and Larks sleep types: the Owls tend to like going to bed later and rising later while Larks are the early to bed/early to rise types. If you are strongly one type or the other this might influence your timing preferences however, as I also mentioned, most of us can flex our style and adopt a bit of both traits.

You've probably heard the saying *'Early to bed, early to rise'* and I believe there is some truth in it. If we can begin to prepare ourselves to sleep well before midnight (between 10 to 11pm say) we stand a better chance of getting good, deep, restorative sleep. Also, don't forget that your deepest sleep actually occurs an hour or so after falling asleep and so you can really optimise the quality of this vital sleep stage by going to bed at a reasonable hour.

The timing rule is particularly important with my clients or patients who have been suffering from very disrupted sleep and are trying to re-establish a normal sleep cycle. I encourage them to follow this rule even if they aren't feeling particularly sleepy (fear of lying in bed *not* sleeping can often mask genuine feelings of tiredness). I get them to follow their wind down routines and then, to think about *resting* rather than actually sleeping. Getting my clients to start preparing to rest and sleep during this time sets them up to get better deep sleep later on as the natural rhythm of sleep is established.

The timing rule also applies to the time you wake up and get out of bed. James is a recovering alcoholic who is doing well on his programme but still struggles with his sleep. Part of the problem for him lies in the timing of his sleep. He goes to bed too late around 1 or 2am, rises between 11 and 12pm and often has a long nap in the afternoon. He actually has what is called *Circadian Rhythm Sleep Disorder* in which his sleep cycle has been shifted forward. We have done some work on changing the timing of his sleep – he now gets into bed around 11pm, reads for 20 minutes or so before turning the light out and his alarm goes off at 7.30am. Initially he found this quite hard but after a few weeks of the new 'routine' he is sleeping better and feeling much more energised.

There are some exceptions to this rule of timing and these are:

If you are a Martini sleeper (of course!)
If you've got something better to do – we are social animals after all!
Or if you've been using the tools I've recommended so far and your sleep has been beautifully restored and you are totally unfazed by the odd night of disrupted sleep.

In other words, *this may be the tool you need to apply with some discipline in the initial stages of restoring your sleep patterns.*

Nuts and Bolts 4: Bed comfort

Again, this comes down to personal preference and a case of exploring what really works for you.

So think about your bed right now. Close your eyes and imagine it. Do you conjure up images of cosiness, support and comfort? Does it make you want to sleep in it? If not, what can you do to make it more enticing? I recently had a client who came to see me with classic Tired but Wired sleep, her mind racing as soon as she got into bed. She works in a Call Centre in a complaints team and deals with irate customers all day. Her job, not surprisingly, is stressful and tiring. When I asked her to think about her bed, the first thing that popped into her head was the word 'angry' – her bed linen was burgundy coloured and although of good quality, it didn't make her feel serene and peaceful which is precisely what she needed after an 'angry' day at the call centre. Once she had made this connection, she immediately changed the colours in her sleep environment and immediately started feeling more calm and relaxed at night time.

Do you think this sleep tool is one that you need to use? Think about your sleep environment – which side of the bed do you prefer to sleep on? And how many pillows do you prefer? What about the thickness of your duvet and softness of your mattress? It really is worth making the time and investment to ensure you get this right to ensure that your bed is your haven for rest and not the place where you spend hours tossing and turning trying to get comfortable.

The last three **Nuts and Bolts** tools are about your relationship with time and they work in quite different ways.

Nuts and Bolts 5: Switch it off!

Perhaps another tool from the school of the blindingly obvious but if you want to get good sleep then you've got to switch your electronic equipment off! This includes mobile phones, BlackBerries, the television, your computer and computer games. Many of my patients with sleep problems have an unhealthy relationship with their gadgets – they can't let go of them, they can't switch them off, and they actually sleep with them beside their bed or actually under their pillow! Research is currently being conducted into the harmful effects of electromagnetic radiation on the brain. While the results are still somewhat inconclusive, it does make good sense to have all such devices switched off and away from your place of rest – especially if you are having problems sleeping. Ask yourself, do I really need to have this switched on? Do I really need to know who is emailing me or what the share prices are at 3am? Some of my clients reply 'yes' very emphatically – they find it hard to see that they have a choice or that the choices they are making are disrupting their sleep.

Technology is a wonderful thing but let's not forget who's the boss here . . .

Nuts and Bolts 6: Time management

I'm sure there are times when you wake up thinking about things that you need to do the next day. You wake up suddenly and that email that you meant to send before you left work is at the front of your mind and not only can you not let go of it, but other worries and 'have to do's' start crowding into your head and stop you falling asleep. Before long, you're wide awake and thinking about sending yourself a voicemail reminder! This is a common source of sleep disruption and one that fortunately can be easily rectified.

Firstly, let's try to understand what is happening. As I mentioned in part 1 your working memory accumulates information throughout the day and then goes offline and files the information during the day when (or if) you take breaks and when you sleep. When you don't take breaks the working memory accumulates information and there is more filing to be done during your REM sleep. So you are most likely to wake up worrying about unfinished business during your REM sleep and often in the early hours of the morning when your sleep depth becomes shallower.

So what is the solution? First of all, try to take more breaks during the day – *build more rest into your day* to allow your brain important consolidation time but also, *practice good time management*. In its simplest form this means keep an organised list-writing system that you update *at the end of the day*. It is essential that you do this at the *end* of the day as this will ensure that you are actually unloading the working memory before you go to sleep. Writing your list at the beginning of the day actually keeps the information in your working memory all night – where it is more likely to wake you up and disrupt your sleep.

Sally is a busy secretary who works for three demanding lawyers at a City law firm. Her workload is extremely high and she works long hours. She enjoys her work and is good at it but often wakes several times throughout the night worrying about things she needs to do the next day. She keeps a pad and pencil by her bed and writes things down but then finds it difficult to get back to sleep. I asked Sally about how she manages her time. 'Oh I have got a very good memory – it's all up here,' she said pointing to her head. Sally did have a good memory and she was writing lists but her time management system was clearly not helping her sleep. 'I write my lists first thing in the morning on coloured sticky notes which are stuck to my computer. I remove them throughout the day as I get through my

tasks.' I asked Sally to close her eyes and think about her working space and how it felt to her. Did it make her feel in control?
She came up with two words 'multicoloured mayhem!' Sally
started writing lists in a notebook at the end of the day. Her
sleep problems disappeared.

This is one of my favourite tips because it is so easy to do
and it makes such a dramatic difference – and very quickly. You
could almost consider this time management tip to be part of
your pre-sleep wind down routine even though you do it earlier in the day, perhaps before you leave work. The key message
you are sending to your brain is, 'I know what I need to do
tomorrow so I can leave it behind me now.' This is a message
about feeling secure and in control and don't forget, we are
much more likely to sleep well when we feel safe.

Nuts and Bolts 7: Stop clock watching!

This 'time management' tip is quite different from the previous
one and is about your relationship with time. Do you remember waking up last night? And if so, do you remember what
time it was when you woke up? I have patients and clients who
could probably plot complex graphs detailing when they woke
up, when they fell asleep again, how many hours of sleep they
got – they are incredibly preoccupied with *checking the time*.
The problem with this particular habit is that it increases attentional bias. You may remember earlier we looked at how sleep
problems can arise and we end up *trying too hard* to get to sleep.
If you are a sensitive sleeper, checking the time can be very disruptive to your sleep. Every time you check, your brain starts
calculating and risk-assessing and then all of the worries of the
day start crowding in and you're wide awake.

The problem with all of this calculation and assessing is that
it stops you navigating through the hynagogic trance state and

back into sleep. It is *completely normal to wake during the night.*
What is not normal is to then adopt behaviours that stop you
getting back to sleep – such as checking the time.

Does this ring any bells? If it does then stop checking the
time every time you wake up! Some of my clients – usually
Martini sleepers – say to me 'I love looking at the clock and
knowing that I've got another hour or so in bed'. For them,
clock-watching isn't a problem and they are able to slide effortlessly back into sleep. For others, if clock watching is *not working
for you* then you need to stop doing it! It's as simple as that.
Strangely, even though it is simple and effective, some of my
patients struggle with it. 'I just need to know the time!' One of
my patients, a chronic fatigue sufferer, said this to me recently.
This particular lady had *three alarm clocks* in her room just in
case she 'slept through her alarm' (although she never did). I
had to work hard to convince her to relinquish her grip on
needing to know the time and when she did, she began to find
it easier to return to sleep when she woke up.

Nuts and Bolts Tools in action:
How Tony used the Nuts and Bolts Tools
To Sleep in Hotel Rooms

Tony, a busy and successful marketing director for an IT firm,
enjoys his job and the travel that it entails. He makes several
business trips each month often to far-flung destinations like
Australia and the Far East. His problem is that he can't sleep
when he gets to his hotel room. It became clear after our first
session together that Tony needed to use some Nuts and Bolts
tools and he set about making the following changes:

- He travels with small pictures of his family to place on the
  hotel bedside table.

- He clears away all visible signs of work when he has finished his day's work – briefcase, laptop and papers in the cupboard. Work clothes ready and hung in the wardrobe.
- He tries to fit in at least 30 minutes of exercise in the hotel gym to help him wind down before his dinner.
- He chooses a light meal from the room service menu or eats lightly if he is dining out with clients. He avoids alcohol.
- He arranges the bed so that he is sleeping on his preferred side of the bed and removes any excess pillows and covers.
- He arranges the curtains and drapes so that the right amount of light enters the room in the morning.
- He experiments with the air-conditioning settings so that the temperature is just right for him.
- He avoids watching TV in bed.
- He organises his morning wake-up call and then covers up all visible time-keeping devices. He switches off his BlackBerry.
- He calls his family before he settles down to read a book that is light-hearted, uplifting and easy to read.
- He uses a breathing technique to help in slide effortlessly into sleep. (You will learn about this when you get to the Power Tools).

Now you might be thinking, 'That's quite a list! How does he remember to do all of that?' Well it took Tony a little while to work out exactly what was right for him and then he just set about replacing some of his previous unhelpful sleep rituals with the ones that give him the sleep that not only sets him up for a good day's work but, most importantly, delivers him back to his own home with energy and in good spirits. Tony's routines are now so hard-wired into his behaviour that they are second nature and he doesn't really have to give them too much thought – they just happen automatically.

What changes do you need to make to your pre-sleep routine and sleep environment? Which tools do you think you need to use? Don't forget, this is personal so use your inner voice to help you select and experiment with the tools that will really work for you.

REMEMBER:
- Your external environment is key to your sleep – pay attention to what makes you feel safe and secure.
- Pay attention to sounds, sights, smells, temperature, the feelings that your sleep space invoke in you.
- Develop and customise your pre-sleep wind down routine so that it becomes second nature for you.
- Practice good time management so that you can leave work out of your bedroom and sleep.
- Avoid checking the time during the night if this stops you getting back to sleep.
- Use your routine with discipline particularly when you travel or feel stressed.
- Aim to use each tool for at least 21 days to create a sustainable change.

CHAPTER 7

The Basic Tools

Earlier on in Part 1 of my book, we looked at the science behind sleep and the stages and cycles of sleep. As I am sure you have gathered, the process of sleep is quite complex and intricately engineered. Your brain produces a delicate balance of hormones that tell the body that it is time to rest and sleep: But as I have said before *sleep problems are created well before you get into bed.* Everything that you do during the day influences your physiology, biochemistry and therefore the way you will sleep.

These are some of the Basic Tools that are most effective for creating the right internal environment for sleep:

Nutrition
Avoiding stimulants
Hydration
Exercise and movement

Basic Tool 1: Nutrition: The 6 Steps to Good Sleep

Very early in my career I noticed that poor nutrition played a significant role in creating bad sleep. I have no doubt that this also played a major part in my own sleep problems as my student years were fuelled mainly by caffeine, nicotine, alcohol and chocolate! I spent hundreds of hours assessing the physiology of my clients and talking to them about their health. Time and again I noticed that the people who talked about poor sleep were the ones who had bad eating habits. I then noticed a similar pattern when I started working with my patients at the hospital.

While this is not meant to be a textbook of nutrition, there are a few changes that you may need to make to your eating pattern – and they might be relatively small – that could significantly improve your sleep.

STEP 1: EAT BREAKFAST WITHIN 30 MINUTES OF WAKING UP

This is the first and most important element of your 'sleep nutrition' and I can't over-emphasise how important it is. Virtually *every* client or patient that I see with a combination of sleep problems and fatigue is falling short on using this tool – they don't eat breakfast! Or at least, they might eat breakfast but it happens 1-2 hours after they get out of bed. Often they don't feel like eating breakfast because it actually makes them feel nauseous and they just don't have the appetite. Also, they skip breakfast because they never have the time for it as they are always running late. And why is this? Because they constantly press the snooze button eking out every last second of sleep because they haven't slept well and are so tired. With many of these individuals I also see, as part of this pattern, a strong reliance on caffeine or nicotine to rev them up during the day, and alcohol to help them wind down at the end of the day.

Does any of this ring bells with you?

If it does, don't worry. If you take the breakfast tool and start using it regularly – *every day for the next 21 days* – you will really start to notice a difference in your energy levels and then your sleep.

When we eat breakfast – and this means consuming food within 30-40 minutes of rising – we send an important message to the brain that there is adequate food in our environment. When we don't eat, this sends a simple message to the brain that there is no food available. That is, we are living in famine conditions.

The biochemistry of being well-fed is very different from that of the famine state and is particularly relevant to how you are going to sleep at the end of the day. When we eat healthily, and the first step is eating breakfast, we are starting to create the perfect internal chemistry for optimal sleep. In the well-fed state our metabolism is higher as we are using up our energy stores (so we feel more energised), blood sugar control is more stable, we have the resources to make the mood hormone serotonin (so we feel better), and we have the resources to make the sleep hormone melatonin at the end of the day when the light drops – so we sleep better!

In the famine state our internal chemistry is completely wrong for sleep. The adrenal glands produce adrenaline to give us the energy to survive in the absence of any food, we conserve our energy stores to help us survive until we next get food, we start to rely on adrenaline-like substances to give us energy – caffeine and refined sugars, we don't invest our energy and biochemical resources in any non-essential physiological processes such as sleep. *This is the physiology of being Tired but Wired!*

Unfortunately, because it may seem like a minor change, one could easily underestimate the value of this particular tool – but believe me, I have seen the positive results time and time again. Now every time I mention the word 'breakfast' to a group of patients or clients I brace myself for the storm of protests and excuses! Here are just a few of them:

- 'I'm never hungry in the morning. In fact, the thought of eating makes me feel sick!' – I have heard this many times from non-breakfast eaters. If you don't normally eat breakfast first thing, then your metabolism is not primed for it and you may feel a bit queasy. The important thing is to start small – perhaps a glass of smoothie, or a small banana or half a piece of toast. Over time (usually 3-4 weeks or so), your physiology will start to adjust and you will notice you wake up feeling hungry.
- 'I don't have the time to have breakfast' – another popular excuse and I heard this just recently from a lady who not only gave her children breakfast before they went to school but managed to down 4 cups of tea while doing so! I'm not talking about sitting down to a luxury three-course meal but just eating something small and nutritious as quickly and efficiently as you can even if you are on the go. I love sitting down to a big breakfast, with the family and the papers on a Sunday morning but during the week breakfast eating is fast, functional and an essential investment towards my energy for the day and good sleep at night.
- 'Eating breakfast will make me gain weight' – some of my clients don't eat breakfast as a means of controlling their weight. The interesting point is that it is often my non-breakfast eating clients who have weight problems. Eating a healthy, well-balanced breakfast (see table below) can

actually help you to lose weight because it kick-starts your metabolism for the day and keeps it high throughout the day.

• 'It makes me feel more hungry during the day' – Bingo! This means it is working and your metabolism is being fired up. The trick is to then snack healthily throughout the day to keep fuelling your metabolism.

Natural probiotic yoghurt with muesli and fruit

Porridge topped with nuts and seeds or ground almonds

Milk shake made with frozen fruit, milk, yoghurt and vanilla essence

Scrambled eggs on wholemeal toast

Poached egg on wholemeal toast

Baked beans on wholemeal toast with sprinkling of grated cheese

The healthy cooked breakfast – Poached egg, grilled tomatoes, mushrooms, sausage

---

Healthy Breakfasts for Good Sleep

STEP 2: SNACK HEALTHILY BETWEEN MEALS

This follows on from what I have said about the effects of eating breakfast, stabilising your blood sugar and minimising adrenaline production.

This may be very contrary to what you have been told in the past – that we shouldn't snack between meals but actually I have found that this is one of the ways in which we can adapt better to living and working in our fast-paced society in which the demands placed on our energy may be huge and relentless. Also, for many of us our meals are often snatched and inadequate at meeting these demands both in terms of content and timing.

Aim for a small mid-morning and mid-afternoon snack of about 120 calories or so. This might be a small pot of yoghurt and a piece of fruit, a small handful of nuts and seeds, a small sandwich with lean meat or a couple of rice crackers with peanut butter or hummus. Ideally, the snack would contain a small amount of protein (as do each of these examples) – this provides the amino acids that are essential for melatonin production at night time.

STEP 3: AVOID EATING HEAVILY BEFORE BED

After having eaten, try to allow yourself at least 90 minutes before going to bed. I am sure you have heard this many times but a heavy meal before sleeping is not only disruptive to your sleep but also bad for your health. Most of those calories will go straight into your fat stores (particularly around your abdomen) especially if they come from highly refined and processed foods.

STEP 4: HAVE A SMALL PRE-BEDTIME SNACK

This might seem like a contradiction to the previous tool but it isn't: this is for those of you who wake up during the night feeling hungry. Do you have a fast metabolism? Is your weight well controlled? Do you do a lot of exercise? If the answer to each of these questions is 'yes', then this may be the tool for you. Again, flying in the face of what you may have been told about eating before you go to bed, I have found that this really does work for some of my clients. But do be mindful of the calories – I really do mean a *small* snack. This might be one slice of toast with honey, or a small bowl of cereal with milk, or some warm milk or hot chocolate.

STEP 5: EAT TRYPTOPHAN-RICH FOODS

Tryptophan is the amino acid or protein building block that helps you to make serotonin and melatonin. Certain foods are rich in tryptophan and can therefore help you to sleep better. These foods include lettuce, all poultry, tuna, milk, yoghurt and eggs. Many healthy foods contain tryptophan so it is important to follow a well-balanced, healthy diet and to pay particular attention to your *pattern* of eating so that you are maintaining a good regular intake of tryptophan throughout the day.

STEP 6: TAKE A GOOD MULTIVITAMIN SUPPLEMENT

If your diet may be lacking in all of the vital ingredients and micronutrients, I consider that taking a basic multivitamin supplement is a good insurance policy. There is also some evidence that taking magnesium supplements can help to improve your sleep quality, particularly if you suffer from restless legs syndrome.

Basic Tool 2: Avoid Stimulants

I have already described many case studies in which stimulants – nicotine, alcohol, caffeine, refined sugars, recreational drugs – played a significant role in creating a fatigue cycle and poor sleep. Stimulants disrupt the internal chemistry that is essential for good sleep

CUT DOWN ON CAFFEINE

I am sure you have got the message about how bad caffeine is for your sleep. Some of us, myself included, are more sensitive to caffeine than others. A client recently told me that he was drinking in excess of fifteen strong cups of coffee a day and was sleeping like a log! But he looked like death – his skin was grey with deep, dark circles under his eyes – and he was exhausted during the day.

The half-life of caffeine – the time taken to remove half of the caffeine from your body – of caffeine is about 5hrs. This means if you have a cup of coffee or tea at around 5pm you will still have half of it in your blood stream at 10pm. This may not be enough to make you feel like going out to a party but it will affect your sleep. Caffeine also stops the liver from breaking down adrenaline so it actually adds to the feeling of being tired but wired and stressed.

How does caffeine affect your sleep? The effects of caffeine on sleep are quite clear-cut: it usually delays sleep onset, shortens overall sleep time, and reduces the depth of sleep. It does this by blocking the actions of the 'sleep molecule' I mentioned previously, adenosine. When adenosine stops working the action of stimulating hormones such as adrenaline and dopamine increases. So after consuming caffeine, sleepers are more easily aroused, move more during sleep, and report a reduction in the quality of sleep. The research indicates that the effects of caffeine on dreaming are less clear however my clients tell me (and this has also been my personal experience) that their dreams are more vivid, disturbing and disruptive. You will learn more about this when you get to Chapter 11.

Take a look at **The Caffeine Buzzometer** below to help you assess how much caffeine you are consuming every day. This shows the approximate amounts of caffeine in some popular drinks. You should aim to have no more than 200-300mg/caffeine per day and even less than this if your sleep is a problem.

So a few rules about caffeine:

- Avoid any caffeine after 2pm (this includes tea, coffee, coca cola and many 'energy' drinks)
- Avoid having more than 2 or 3 cups of tea or coffee per day
- If you are drinking more than 2 or 3 cups of tea or coffee per day, cut back gradually, drink more water and start snacking healthily to maintain your energy levels.

The more caffeine you consume, the greater tolerance you develop not only to the caffeine itself but to your body's own natural stimulants so you start needing more and more stimulants to feel normal and motivated. The adrenal glands work harder to produce the adrenaline and then eventually give up resulting in adrenal exhaustion – chronic fatigue, apathy, depression and an inability to cope or care.

	Caffeine/mg
Cup of tea	40–80
Cup of instant coffee	80–100
Starbucks Grande cappuccino	350–450
Can of Red Bull	80
Can of Relentless (16.9 fl oz)	160
Green tea	20–30
Decaf coffee	10–20
Coffee (espresso, latte, cappuccino)	80
Hot chocolate drink	10–20
Coca cola (12 fl oz)	45
Diet coke (12 fl oz)	45
Proplus tablet	50

The Caffeine Buzzometer

AVOID ALCOHOL, NICOTINE AND RECREATIONAL DRUGS

For some of my clients an over-reliance on caffeine is also tied up with excessive alcohol consumption and even drug addictions. Of course, disrupted sleep and insomnia is always part and parcel of this messy picture. I have had some of my best results with clients with addictions who are stuck in an extreme fatigue cycle relying heavily on alcohol, drugs and caffeine to either energise them or help them relax. Once I can show them how to take small steps towards breaking the patterns they have become stuck in they revel in the wonderful feelings of living with their body's own natural internal chemistry.

As with caffeine, we all have variable tolerances to alcohol and the bottom line is that any amount of alcohol will affect the architecture of your sleep – the amount and efficiency of your REM sleep and the quality of your deep sleep. However, it is very pleasant to share a nice bottle of wine with friends and I certainly allow myself the occasional indulgence if I feel that I can afford the less than optimal sleep I might have as a result. In other words, I avoid alcohol if I need to be firing on all cylinders the next day. The bottom line is if your insomnia has become severe and you are trying to rebuild your connection with sleep, it would be advisable to steer clear of alcohol until the improvements to your sleep have become well established.

Like caffeine, the effects of alcohol on sleep are also quite clear. Alcohol has a dual effect and is both a relaxant and a stimulant so it might help initiate sleep – in other words, you fall asleep quickly (or pass out, in the case of some of my clients) but the stimulant effects kick in before you complete the sleep cycle and deep sleep quality is reduced. Alcohol also affects the vital 'filing' processes that I have described earlier – imagine having a drunk filing clerk in your office trying to 'help' you with your piles of filing. Large amounts of alcohol are also likely to cause heavy snoring and other breathing difficulties.

Nicotine is a stimulant and it enhances the effect of adrenaline. So if you smoke for the relaxant effect, do bear in mind that it will disrupt your sleep. Some of my clients have been smoking for years and don't really notice any effect on their sleep until they quit smoking and then realise how much more energy they have and how much better is their quality of sleep. Nicotine can also exacerbate certain sleep disorders such as restless legs syndrome and periodic limb movement disorder.

Basic Tool 3: Hydration

Hydration is so important that it deserves its own compartment in the toolkit. As with many of my 'quick and easy' tools this is one that can yield a huge return in terms of improving your sleep and your energy levels so please don't be tempted to ignore it.

When my daughter was a baby, one of the first challenges that was presented to me as a new mother was how often should I feed her, how much food and liquid did she need? It was a particularly hot summer and I had to work hard at making sure she was well hydrated. If I got it right, she slept beautifully. If I didn't she became cranky and her sleep was more fitful. As adults, our demands for hydration may not be as sensitive as a baby's, but we too are dependent upon water to create that ideal internal sleep chemistry, particularly as an adult human being consists of 70-80% water.

So how much should we be drinking? As with all of these tools, it is a case of working out what is exactly right for us. I recommend that my clients start by aiming for 1 litre per day and then gradually increasing up to 2 to 3 litres per day – sipping throughout the day. This includes diluted fruit squashes or juices, vegetable juices and herbal teas but not caffeinated beverages. It also includes the water in your food although this is less easy to quantify.

And how will you know if you are well hydrated? As a rule of thumb, the best way to tell is by the colour of your urine, which should be pale yellow, and without odour. This test will tell you if 1litre/day is enough for you or 3litres/day.

A few rules about hydration – aim to do this for 21 days, don't drink all of your daily quota in one go – this may be uncomfortable and you will end up passing most of it out as urine – sip throughout the day, if you haven't drunk much water for years, your kidneys may initially protest and you may end up needing to go to the toilet a little more often. This will settle down as walls of you bladder gain muscle tone and become used to holding more liquid. In some respects, this can be a difficult tool to use because *it's almost too easy* but try it and you will really begin to notice a difference to the quality of your sleep – it will feel more refreshing, you will wake up feeling more alert and energised and you may even be less inclined to keep pressing the snooze button.

Basic Tool 4: Exercise and Movement: Creating the Right Activity/Rest Balance

There is a very simple but powerful link between movement and sleep – when we achieve the right amount of movement and exercise throughout the day, we sleep better. Don't forget this is all about creating the right internal chemistry for your sleep and movement is an important part of the equation. Briefly, I mentioned that throughout the day, when you move you produce a chemical called adenosine. The build up in the levels of adenosine is the stimulus to stop adrenaline (and other stimulating hormones) being produced and initiate the bio-chemical changes necessary for sleep.

Apart from adenosine production there are other reasons that movement makes us sleep better:

WHY EXERCISE?

Exercise helps us to shift excess weight and improve breathing.
It boosts the production of hormones that make us feel relaxed and mellow such as endorphins and serotonin.
It rids the body of hormones that make us feel anxious and 'wired' such as adrenaline.
It enables us to switch off – the working memory goes offline.
It helps to open up another part of the brain involving creativity and problem-solving.

And it's not just about sleep. From an evolutionary perspective, human beings are built for movement – it is hard-wired into our physiology as a survival mechanism – and it is highly unnatural and unhealthy to be sedentary.

Every human body has its own unique activity/rest balance – this means that in order to stay in good health and sleep well we need to work out how much rest we need and how much activity we need. In the next chapter, we will look at Rest as one of the Power Tools. But, for now, let's think about movement and exercise.

Some people need more exercise than others but we *all* need movement to help us sleep well. However, many of my clients are not sleeping well, are exhausted and don't exercise because they feel they don't have the energy. Many of them are stuck in the fatigue cycle I have already described and they need to take small steps towards getting their energy levels up so that they can start becoming more active. These small steps usually involve using the first two basic tools – nutrition and hydration – before we can get them exercising.

It can be hard to contemplate exercising when you feel exhausted but I would like you to start thinking a little differently about your energy levels. It may sound odd but sometimes we may think we have no energy but in fact, what we actually have is *compressed* energy. Let me explain.

Have you even noticed how tiring *sitting* can be? A few days ago I was on a business trip that entailed spending six hours sitting on trains. At the end of the day I was very tired (and a little grumpy) and had to drag myself out for a 30 minute run. At the start of the run I felt heavy and tired, my breathing laboured and I wondered why I was doing this to myself. And then 10 minutes into my run my energy had picked up, my breathing had settled and I starting feeling like myself again. Most importantly, I returned home after my run with my energy and spirit lifted and that night I slept like a baby.

Lack of movement built up over a period of time can be exhausting and after a long period of sitting, the last thing you may feel like doing is actually moving because it feels as if you have no energy. However, it may be more a case of your energy becoming 'compressed' or 'stuck'. In scientific terms it might be more accurate to describe your energy as being in the form of 'potential' or stored energy. As you may know, the energy of movement is called 'kinetic energy'. Let's try this exercise to 'de-compress' your energy or, in other words, to convert your potential energy into kinetic energy:

I'd like you to put this book down and now just start rubbing your hands together. Rub them as fast and as vigorously as you can, you should start to feel heat being generated between your palms. You might even feel tension moving up your arms and into your shoulders. Now I want you to stop, shake your hands out quickly and then drop them into your lap.

What did you feel? You might have felt heat and tingling. Try it once more and notice the effect that just this tiny amount of movement has on your body. Do you feel slightly more energised in your body? If so, you have very effectively transformed potential (stored) energy into kinetic (movement) energy. In other words, when we move we feel more energised. We create the right activity/rest balance for deep, peaceful sleep.

So do you think this is the tool for you? Is your daily life and routine too sedentary? Do you need to move more to correct your activity /rest balance?

WHAT TYPE OF EXERCISE?

A well-balanced exercise programme should include exercises for stamina, strength and suppleness. Stamina comes from doing aerobic exercise such as jogging, cycling, swimming or fast walking and should form the core of your exercise programme. Weight training exercises will help you to build strength and muscle tone as well as improving your body's ability to burn calories efficiently. Suppleness and flexibility can be gained by simply stretching in front of the television or doing yoga or pilates.

HOW MUCH EXERCISE?

To get really fit, the government recommendations are that you need to do more than half an hour of gentle daily activity. The American College of Sports Medicine (ACSM) recommends moderately intense cardiovascular exercise (to the point where you break into a sweat and can talk) 30 minutes a day, five days a week, or vigorously intense cardiovascular exercise (to the point where you are breathless) 20 minutes a day, three days a week. The ACSM also recommends an additional twice weekly weight training programme comprising 8 to 10 strength-training exercises with 8 to 12 repetitions of each.

It is also a good idea to vary your routine. If you do the same workout over and over again, not only will you become bored but also your body is never challenged. It is by challenging your body that you become stronger and fitter.

If you are inactive can you start to take small steps towards making movement an essential part of your life? Can you avoid the lift and start using the stairs, can you start walking to work or at least part of the way, can you join a gym or walking club?

Just one final note about exercise, intense competitive exercise can actually stop you sleeping well – it raises your core temperature and can be over stimulating and, as I have mentioned before, your body temperature is key to you getting good sleep. So if you do indulge in any competitive sport, do be mindful of the need to allow yourself extra time to wind down afterwards. Slow right down and use your nuts and bolts tools to create the transition between activity and rest.

Basic Tools in action: How Lisa used the Basic Tools to improve her sleep

Lisa is a 30yr old mother of three young children. She helps her husband to run their chain of clothes shops, and in her spare time runs a film production studio! Lisa came to see me because she wasn't sleeping well and, not surprisingly, she was exhausted and grumpy with the children. All it took was one session and her sleep, energy levels and mood had significantly improved. All she did was to start eating healthily – she started eating breakfast with the children and having healthy snacks during the day. She also started drinking more water and cut back on caffeine. When she came back to see me for her second session she had started jogging and playing tennis again. These are significant changes and, to her credit, she was very motivated and disciplined to make them – and she really reaped the benefits. I never saw Lisa again – I didn't need to. A simple piece of work with a very happy ending.

You have now been introduced to the full set of basic tools. Which ones do you think you need to start using? Decide what changes you are going to make and when you will start making them. Who can support you in making these changes? Can you maintain these changes for at least 21 days? How will you stop yourself relapsing back into bad habits? How can you keep reminding yourself of your vision for your sleep to stop yourself relapsing?

REMEMBER, BRILLIANT SLEEP CAN BE CREATED BY:

- Good nutritional habits – especially eating breakfast first thing in the morning.
- Steering clear of stimulants such as caffeine, alcohol, and recreational drugs.
- Staying well hydrated.
- Building the right amount of exercise and movement into your day.

CHAPTER 8

Power Tools (I) – Optimal Breathing

Now we come to the first of the power tools:
The Optimal Breathing Technique (OBT).

This tool is the equivalent of the most powerful electrical drill in a builder's toolkit. In the next chapter, you will learn how to refine your use of the Optimal Breathing Technique to optimise the quality of your sleep. But for now, let's focus on the basics . . .

> If you want to sleep brilliantly, you have to learn how to rest and relax brilliantly.

The Art of Relaxation

Many people have lost the art of relaxation and my work often involves educating clients on exactly how to relax. A running coach once gave me a definition of 'relaxation' that has stuck in my mind ever since. He said '*relaxation is the absence of unnecessary effort*'. He was trying to get me to relax so that I could run more effortlessly. But can you see how this definition applies so beautifully to life in general and sleep?

BREATHING – THE KEY TO BEING RELAXED

If you have ever attended a relaxation or yoga class, you will know that the key to being able to relax is through your breathing.

> Deep diaphragmatic breathing prepares the body and mind to rest and relax. Rest and relaxation prepare the body and mind to sleep.

When I explained the science of sleep to you, I mentioned the vagus nerve – that important part of the nervous system that is activated when you breathe deeply and which helps to initiate the relaxation and sleep process. For many of my clients, the key to restoring their sleep is by actually 'retraining' their breathing patterns and thereby firing up the vagus nerve.

As a research scientist, I spent a lot of time studying breathing or respiratory physiology. But when I left the world of theory and research and began working with real human beings I was puzzled by a discrepancy between what I had learnt and researched and what I was measuring and observing.

As I worked with my clients, I became aware that breathing is one of the first aspects of our physiology that is affected when we become tense and anxious. As soon as our brain registers threat, this triggers the release of adrenaline and other stress hormones, the so-called *fight or flight* response. The stress hormones shift our breathing up to the chest area as we try to take in more air and oxygen to give us the energy and momentum to fight or flee from the threat (real or imagined).

If you habitually breathe from your chest you will feel tired and listless as you will only have access to about 20% of your lung capacity so you won't be getting the right amount of oxygen into your lungs. You might find yourself constantly yawning, sighing or even hiccupping as a client did last week! You may experience soreness in your neck and shoulders from having to constantly move the weight of your rib cage, thorax and shoulders. Although this might not sound like a lot of work it can become so when you consider that we breathe 20-25, 000 times per day! Furthermore, breathing from your chest can literally cause you to breathe yourself into a state of anxiety and panic – as you may have witnessed if you've ever seen anyone having a panic attack.

Many factors can cause chest or shallow breathing – excess abdominal weight and lack of exercise, adrenaline and stress, smoking, and even your diet – excessive amounts of caffeine, sugars and even starvation can affect your breathing. Poor posture can also significantly change your breathing (check yours right now). Many of my depressed patients have very poor posture. They often cross their arms in front of their bodies or sit slumped and defeated – both actions cause the diaphragm to become 'blocked' and shift the breathing up into the chest area. Not surprisingly, these patients find themselves constantly sighing, feeling exhausted and suffering from tightness in their neck, shoulders and upper back.

So clearly, chest breathing is not conducive to creating brilliant sleep. So what is? Of course, the answer is deep belly breathing. I call this *Optimal Breathing.*

The Optimal Breathing Technique (OBT): 4 Steps to Relaxation and Sleep

Notice your breathing
Open up your posture
Deepen your breath
Slow down your breathing

I call this the NODS technique. Practised regularly, it will have you nodding off in no time at all!

STEP ONE – NOTICE YOUR BREATHING

For the next twenty to thirty seconds I simply want you to sit comfortably and just observe your breathing. Don't try to control or change anything about your breathing. Just allow it to follow its own natural rhythm. You might find it easier to concentrate if you close your eyes and bring your focus inwards.

Where is your breathing coming from? Is your belly moving? Your chest and shoulders? Are they are both moving? Is your breathing shallow or deep? Is it rapid or slow? Remember, don't try to control or change your breathing in any way at all. Simply pay attention and notice.

And now open your eyes. What did you notice? What did you feel? You might have noticed:

Your chest was moving or
Your belly was moving or
Both areas were moving.

STEP TWO: OPEN UP YOUR BREATHING

I now want you to repeat the above exercise but first I want you to make a few small changes to your posture.

Sit comfortably and place both feet on the floor about hip width apart (I call this **Grounding**).

Straighten up your back, 'unkink' your spine, imagine you have a string attached to the top of your head, pulling you up and elongating your spine (I call this **Centering**).

Relax your hands into your lap and drop your shoulders.

Raise or lower your chin so that it is exactly level with the floor.

Finally, press your tongue up against the roof of your mouth (there is no exact science about how you do this and you can do it with your mouth closed).

Now that you have made these postural changes, close your eyes again and notice your breathing for 20 seconds or so. Does anything feel different now that you have made some changes to your posture and placed your tongue on the roof of your mouth?

You should notice how: Opening up your posture in this way can help to shift your breathing down to your belly.

STEP THREE: DEEPEN YOUR BREATHING

Remain seated, feet firmly planted on the floor, grounded and cen-tred. Close your eyes and focus inwards, but this time focus specifically on your out-breath or exhalation. As before, don't try to control or change your breathing. Simply follow your breath and when you are ready **exhale as completely as you can** – breathe out just a little bit more, and then just a little bit more until it feels as if you have completely emptied your lungs. Now notice the 'tug' of your diaphragm as you breathe in more fully and more deeply. You may have also noticed that your belly 'domed' outwards as you breathed in more deeply.

Try this again. Breathe out as much as you can – don't force it but try to gently empty your lungs as completely as you can. And again, feel the tug of your diaphragm, and the doming of your belly as your lungs completely refill themselves. Now return to your own natural pattern of breathing.

You should notice how:

- The key to deepening your breathing is to actually focus on *exhaling*. In response you will breathe in more deeply.
- Your abdominal muscles are your respiratory mus-cles – they dome out as you breathe in and pull in towards your spine as you breathe out.

STEP FOUR: SLOW YOUR BREATHING

You may have noticed right at the beginning of this exercise that your breathing was shallow and rapid. We are now going to work on slowing it down by building some pauses in between your in and out breaths.

As before, remain seated, feet firmly planted on the floor, grounded and centred. Place your tongue on the roof of your mouth. Close your eyes and focus inwards. Observe your breathing. Begin to deepen your breath by prolonging your exhalation by a few seconds; notice the deepening of your inhalation.

After you next exhale, **pause** briefly for a few seconds if you can, just remain there and be still. Now breathe in and, again, pause for a few seconds.

Try this again,

Prolong your exhalation _ pause briefly _ deepen your inhalation_ pause briefly _exhale_ pause _ inhale _ pause

Have you got the hang of this? You don't need to prolong every exhalation and deepen every inhalation. The trick is to do this for the first few breaths just to 're-route' your breathing and then just let your breathing take over. Hopefully you noticed that by building pauses in between your in and out breaths, your breathing began to slow down.

You should notice how:

> • You can slow your breathing down by pausing momentarily after exhaling and after inhaling.

IF THIS TOOL DIDN'T WORK FOR YOU

Some people find it very hard to use this technique. Although it should come naturally, they have spent so many years breathing badly that this breathing technique is completely alien to them.

Another reason why this might not have worked is if you simply weren't using your abdominal muscles and this might happen if you were holding your belly in tightly. I was recently making a short film about the Optimal Breathing Technique and one of the film crew, a very attractive lady wearing a beautiful figure-hugging suit, volunteered to be the guinea pig for the shoot. So we sat down together and I began to talk her through the Optimal Breathing Technique. But she just couldn't do it! She was holding her stomach and belly in so tightly that she couldn't engage the lower part of her lungs – all of her breathing came from her chest. The harder she tried the more her chest and shoulders moved and the more stressed she became. In the end she had to abandon the exercise and we had to find another willing victim.

> So in order to breathe optimally you need to let go, relax your abdominal muscles and allow your belly to get involved.

If you found it hard to do this exercise, you can try this technique *lying down on the floor* so that gravity helps to engage your diaphragm and your abdominal muscles will naturally be more relaxed. If you have a bad back, please be careful how you do this and you may need to use cushions and blankets to support your back. Lie down and raise your legs so that they are resting on the edge of your bed or chair, or even up a wall if you are very flexible.

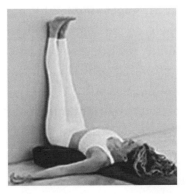

Figure 9: Optimal breathing while lying down

Now that you are in this lying position go through the stages of the **NODS** technique:

Notice your breathing – place your tongue on the roof of your mouth, close your eyes, bring your attention within

Open up your breathing – in this case, your posture will already be open, so just focus on your belly and make sure that your shoulders are relaxed and down

Deepen your breathing by prolonging your exhalation

Slow your breathing by building in brief pauses after your exhalation and inhalation

Can you now feel your breathing shifting from your chest and into your belly? Can you feel your breathing deepening and slowing down?

In case you were wondering why I asked you to place your tongue on the roof of your mouth, there is apparently an 'acupressure point' on the roof of the mouth that when stimulated, helps to switch on the vagus nerve. This little trick is used by martial artists to help create a grounded and relaxed state of focus. This technique is also recommended for use during labour. I have a notion that babies and little children are actually stimulating this pressure point when they latch on to their mother's breast or suck their thumb or dummy – it simply helps them to feel relaxed and calm!

A Habit for Life

So to start retraining your breathing using this essential sleep tool I want you to practise it as often as you can. Do it right now! Place your feet on the ground, straighten up, drop your shoulders, bring your chin level to the floor, place your tongue on the roof of your mouth and simply BREEEATHE . . . In fact for the remainder of this chapter pay attention to your posture and breathing. Try to shift it down to your belly, deepen it and slow it right down.

The principle is that you start to train your body and mind to *accept* the state of rest. You hardwire this into your system *during the day* so that your mind and body is receptive to this state when you are preparing to sleep at night. Consider this as the 'warm up' for the big event – i.e. gliding into brilliant sleep at night.

I recently worked with a client who, to my amazement, said she 'didn't have the time to do the breathing 'thing'! True, she was a stressed out mother of three children who spent a lot of time ferrying between school runs and after school activities *and* she was going through a divorce. But the beauty of this technique lies in its simplicity – you can do it anytime and anywhere. You can do it while you are lying in bed, while sitting in a traffic jam, sitting at your desk, eating your meal, standing in a queue at the supermarket, in a meeting . . .

You can do it *right now*.

The challenge of this technique also lies in its simplicity – breathing is mostly automatic and unconscious and so it is easy to forget and revert to your old, non-restful, chest-breathing pattern. So to help you build your sleep-inducing breathing habit I am going to recommend a prescription for how to take your 'breathing medicine'.

> For the next 21 days I want you to *consciously* practise this breathing technique at least 3-5 times per day.

It doesn't really matter how long you do it for although aiming for 3-5 minutes each time would be ideal. The idea is to bring your attention to your breathing and focus on breathing from your belly (i.e. diaphragm) each time – and to aim to do this for the next three weeks.

Now we're all busy people and even finding the time to *remember to breathe* might be challenging. So try to **link the breathing technique with something that you do regularly**. This might be driving to work, or sitting at your desk or while you watch TV. I have a client who is obsessed with checking his BlackBerry for messages (and he has very Tired but Wired sleep). He now associates BlackBerry with Breathe and, not surprisingly, he has become a very efficient 'belly breather'.

Do it whenever you wake up, as you drift off to sleep and then find a few other times throughout the day. You will start to notice that not only does your sleep improve but also your energy levels throughout the day are much better. Obviously when you are in bed you don't have to sit up and put your feet on the ground. But if you can focus on bringing your awareness to breathing from your belly and deepening your breath by prolonging the exhalation, you will notice that this helps you relax and slide into sleep.

In the next chapter you will learn how to apply this technique to calming your mind when you are agitated, help you get to sleep, or get back to sleep if you wake up during the night. But for now, just practice the basics – even while you read you can work on noticing, opening, deepening and slowing down your breath.

REMEMBER:
- The way you breathe is essential to creating a state of relaxation and rest.
- The way you breathe is essential to helping you sleep.
- The Optimal Breathing Tool can be used to create brilliant sleep.
- The Optimal Breathing Tool consists of Noticing, Opening, Deepening and Slowing down your breath.
- Practise regularly for maximum benefit: 3-5 times per day for the next 21 days.

The Optimal Breathing Technique

This technique can be practiced while sitting or lying down.

Notice your breathing – pay attention to the movement of your chest, shoulders, belly while you breathe. Close your eyes and bring your attention inwards. Where is your breathing coming from?

Open up your breathing – straighten up, roll your shoulders back and down, relax your arms and hands, place your tongue on the roof of your mouth. If you are sitting, raise or lower your chin so that it is parallel to the floor.

Deepen your breathing – prolong your exhalation by a few seconds by pulling your belly in towards your spine. Notice the tug of your diaphragm as you breathe back in more deeply and fully.

Slow your breathing down – at the end of each exhalation, pause momentarily.

Figure 10: The Optimal Breathing Technique

CHAPTER 9

Power Tools (II) – Optimal Breathing in Action

You have now learnt how to use what is probably the most important and powerful tool in the toolkit – the Optimal Breathing Technique (OBT).

Now you will learn how to use this technique to cut through some common sleep problems and create brilliant sleep. Just to remind you, these are some of the commonest problems I encounter in my clinic:

Difficulties falling asleep
Difficulties staying asleep
Fear of going to sleep
Racing thoughts and inability to stop thinking
Restlessness

I would recommend that you start with the basic techniques and then move on to the more advanced techniques. By a process of trial and error, you will begin to work out what tools are right for you and when to use them. In order to help you make the right choices, at the end of each technique you will find a set of mini-instructions and contraindications.

Some of the instructions are fairly detailed so you might find it helpful to actually pre-record them and then play them back while you practise the technique or get someone to read them out to you as you practise.

Power Tool 1: Count yourself to sleep

I'm sure you've heard of counting sheep to get to sleep, this is a version of it. Strictly speaking, you're not actually going to count sheep but you are going to *count yourself to sleep.*

You're lying in bed, tired but you can't fall asleep or return to sleep so what do you do? Get as comfortable as you can – you can lie on your back, front or side whatever feels best for you. Bring your attention to your breathing, close your eyes and focus inwards. Simply pay attention to your breathing and notice it. Your mind might be racing around at the speed of knots but just keep following your breathing. For now, don't try to change it – just allow it to follow its own natural rhythm. When you are ready, experiment with deepening your breath by prolonging your exhalation as I described in the previous chapter with the OBT. Slow it down by building in pauses after exhaling and inhaling. Once you have got the hang of this you are ready to start counting. Here's how you do it . . .

When you next exhale, mentally and silently say the word 'ONE'. The trick with this is to repeat the word ONE for the *entire* duration of the exhalation and to mentally say the word as *softly and gently* as you can. Imagine you are putting a baby to sleep!

Now inhale – pause if you need to – and then silently whisper the word 'TWO' as you exhale for the second time. Repeat this until you get to TEN on your tenth exhalation. When you have got to this point, go right back to ONE and start again.

The most important things to remember about this technique are:

* Whisper the numbers mentally and as softly as you can – your 'inner voice' must be like that of a mother soothing a baby to sleep.
* Whisper the numbers for entire duration of the exhalation – so sometimes the word will be long (oooooooooooooone) sometimes shorter (twooooooo) as each breath varies in length.
* Allow your breathing to set the rhythm of the counting – this is not a military exercise and you don't want to be counting to a marching tune!

Let's return to the exercise. Keep breathing and counting. You will get to a point when you either lose track of the next number, start thinking about something else or drift off. *This is meant to happen.* At this point, go right back to the number 1 and start again. It is really important that you get the hang of this and that as soon as you realise you are losing the ability to count, you return to 1 and restart the process of counting to 10. Don't try to be clever and guess the next number! The idea is to bore yourself to sleep by counting.

I call this moment when you 'forget' to count the 'sweet spot' of sleep. Technically it is the intermediate stage between awake and asleep, the trance state that I have referred to previously as the 'hypnagogic trance'. Another indication that you have hit the sweet spot is when your thoughts start to 'distort'

and become somewhat nonsensical. When you have been practising this technique regularly, you will become more adept at
recognising exactly when you get to this point and you can say
to yourself 'Aha! I'm falling asleep!'

I would like you to put the book down and just try this right
now. You might not want to take it to the point where you
actually fall asleep but I just want you to become familiar with
counting with your breathing, softening your inner voice, and
relaxing into the technique. Make sure you have read through
the instructions a few times, understood and practised them
and then you will be ready to use this sleep 'tool' at night.

KEY POINTS:

- You will be aware of thoughts in your head even while
  you breathe and count, just keep coming back to your
  breathing and the numbers.
- This technique may not work for you if your mind is
  really racing and ruminating obsessively on the same
  thoughts. You may end up counting all night, which can
  feel maddening. If this is the case, move on to the next
  tool.

Power Tool 2: Surfing the breath

This technique is somewhat softer than the previous one.
Most of us love the beach and the sea so the idea behind this
tool is for you to create your perfect beach scene and to use
your senses to put this together with the OBT to lull you to
sleep. It is really quite simple and when you get the hang of
it you can be more creative and use your imagination to add
other visuals to it and make it your own. So here's how you
do it . . .

Get comfortable in whatever position feels best for you.

Bring your attention to your breathing and begin using the OBT.

Once you have settled into doing this for a couple of minutes or so, imagine a beach scene. It is important that this beach is just right for you – perfect temperature, the sky is blue with a few fluffy white clouds, the sea is blue-green. Smell the salt in the air. Feel the warmth against your skin. Look at the waves and the surf. Hear the waves as they wash in to the beach and wash back out to sea. Now begin to synchronise the movement of the waves to your breath.

As you breathe in, the waves wash in to the beach. Mentally and softly whisper the word INNNN as the waves wash in.

As you breathe out, the waves wash back out to the sea. Mentally and softly whisper the word OOOOOUT as the waves wash back out.

It is important the waves are synchronised with your breathing (and not the other way around). So some waves will be big, some smaller. Some come in more rapid succession and others take a while to wash in. The waves are following the irregular pattern of your breathing.

Continue surfing your breath and allow yourself to sink deeper and deeper into relaxation with every breath you take.

KEY POINTS:

- You will be aware of thoughts in your head even while you breathe just keep coming back to your breath and the waves.
- Don't forget to make your inner voice soft and soothing.

Power Tool 3: Pre-sleep yoga

These three pre-sleep yoga postures are very simple and can be practised even if you have never done yoga before. There are some contraindications for using these postures so do take a look at the instructions before you attempt them.

CONTRAINDICATIONS

If you have severe back problems or tight leg muscles and hamstrings then you may need to check with your doctor or physiotherapist before using any of these exercises. If you suffer from mild back problems or tightness in your legs you can use the variations on the postures that are given at the end of this section.

These exercises work on several levels: they calm the mind (which is good if your thoughts are racing), they rebalance the nervous system and help to reduce adrenaline levels, they help to activate the vagus nerve and deepen your breathing, and finally, they prepare the mind and body for rest and sleep.

Ideally, you hold each posture in turn, for 3-5 minutes each, before you get into bed. You might even light a candle, use some relaxing aromatherapy oils and even play some relaxing music. The aim is to create a sanctuary of peace and safety.

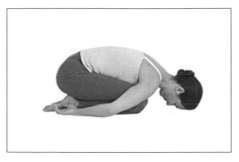

CHILDS POSE

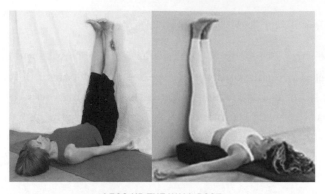

LEGS UP THE WALL POSE

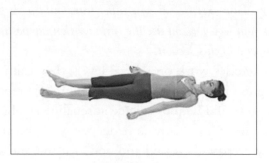

CORPSE POSE

Figure 11: Pre-sleep yoga routine

Move between the postures in the sequence: Childs Pose – Legs up the Wall Pose – Corpse Pose.

In each posture, breathe deeply and allow yourself to completely relax. If thoughts continue to buzz around in your head, don't try to block them but just keep coming back to your breathing. As you did with the 'surfing the breath' technique, you might want to mentally whisper IN/OUT as you breathe.

VARIATIONS FOR MILD BACK PROBLEMS OR TIGHT LEGS

Childs pose – rest your forehead on cushions or a pillow.

Legs up the wall – lie on the floor with your legs over the edge of your bed or sofa. Use cushions and blankets to cushion and support you.

Corpse pose – bend your knees and support your back with blankets and cushions.

KEY POINTS:

Use these techniques as part of your wind down routine before getting into bed.

These routines are particularly helpful if you have been working late.

Use these routines if restless legs stop you falling asleep.

Power Tool 4: Letting Go

In order to be able to sleep, our mind and body must be perfectly relaxed, no tension, no constriction and no holding on. Throughout the day, as we go about our busy lives, our bodies can become more and more tightly 'coiled' like a tight spring. I have patients who come to see me in such a tight state of tension and constriction and, not surprisingly, they can't sleep. Some of them have spent years creating this tension in their bodies and for them, being able to relax and sleep can seem a distant and impossible goal. Very shortly I am going to show you exactly how to begin to 'uncoil' your body but firstly, in case you are in any doubt about how holding on and tension can affect you, I would like you to try the following exercise:

Clench your fists; clench them as hard as you can, until you can see your knuckles turning white, your nails digging into your palms. Clench harder. This should now start to hurt. You may now notice that the tension and pain is spreading up through your forearms, your upper arms, maybe even your shoulders and jaws. This 'clenching' may start to spread to your face as you find yourself biting down hard with your teeth and tensing your jaw muscles. This should now feel very uncomfortable.

And now, just let go. Relax your palms. What can you feel? Perhaps relief at letting go. Warmth flooding your hands as the blood returns. Maybe your hands will now feel lighter, looser somehow. You may find that this release of tension has even spread to your arms, shoulders and face.

I recently asked a client to do this exercise – 17-year-old Sean has had problems sleeping for years. When I asked him how he felt when he unclenched his hands, he said 'light and *relaxed*'. He said the last word with a note of wonder in his voice – as if he couldn't believe that he could possibly *feel* relaxed as he had spent so many years feeling exactly the opposite. Doing this simple exercise reminded him how it felt to be relaxed and, most importantly, that maybe he *could* relax and sleep.

Power Tool 5: Progressive muscle relaxation (PMR)

This exercise works well if your mind is continually running over the events of the day and you just can't let them go. I have also found that this exercise works particularly well for highly driven 'A' types – those who like to be in control, perfectionistic and needing things to be *just so*, are impatient and hate slowing down.

The 'letting go' exercise brings together several of the elements of the previous techniques so it truly is a power tool. It also uses the technique of *progressive muscle relaxation* and so it is particularly good for those of you who store your stress in your muscles and need to let go.

Before you start, prepare your environment to your exact taste – soft lighting, soft music, aromatherapy oils or scented candles.

Lie with your legs up the wall or over the side of a chair/bed. Use cushions or blankets to make yourself more comfortable. Close your eyes and allow your weight to settle and relax into the floor.

Bring your attention to your breathing. Focusing on the movement of your belly and feeling it rise when you breathe in and fall back towards your spine as you breathe out. As you breathe in, mentally repeat IIINNNNNN. As you breathe out repeat OOOUUUTTT. Make your 'inner voice' soft, slow and soothing – as if you are lulling a baby to sleep.

Become aware of the deepening of your out-breath. Try and extend it if you can and notice how your in-breath deepens in response. Notice the slight gap or lull at the end of each breath.

You may notice thoughts, sensations in your body, awareness of sounds – don't try to block them out. Just keep bringing your attention back to following your breathing. Start to become aware of any tension in your body. Scan through from your toes to the top of your head letting go of tension as follows:

Wriggle your toes . . . and relax and let go

Point your toes towards and away from you . . . and relax and let go

Contract your thighs . . . and relax and let go

Squeeze your buttocks . . . and relax and let go

Squeeze your abdominal muscles . . . and relax and let go

Squeeze your shoulders up to your ears . . . and relax and let go

Make fists with your hands, raise them up . . . and relax and let go

Scrunch up your face . . . soften and let go

Relax the space between your eyebrows

Soften your jaw, mouth, cheeks, allow your eyes to roll back into their sockets

Become aware of anywhere else in your body where there is tension and let it go, feel it draining out of your body into the floor. Feel yourself softening, relaxing, allowing your body to melt into the floor.

Follow your breathing – in and out – with every out-breath feeling yourself relaxing deeper and deeper and letting go.

KEY POINT:

You can use this technique as part of your wind down routine before getting into bed or at any time during the day if you find yourself become tense or stressed.

Power Tool 6: Power Napping

We now come to the crème de la crème of power tools. I consider this to be not only incredibly powerful but also amongst my favourite. Throughout history there are many examples of famous inventors, artists and scientists who experimented with their sleep, napped prodigiously and suffered no ill-effects. In fact, they attributed their success to their sleep habits. To name just a few – Leonardo Da Vinci, Thomas Edison, Nikola Tesla,

Salvador Dali, Albert Einstein and Winston Churchill. In fact, I have to confess that I too have become a 'napper' and I attribute much of my good sleep and energy to learning how to rest and nap wherever and whenever I can.

With regular practise you really will find that napping is highly portable and that you can use it to enhance your performance in many areas of your life and not just sleep. Many of my clients use power napping before sport, presentations or important meetings and driving long distances. Most recently, a scientist Olaf Lahl and his team of researchers at the University of Dusseldorf in Germany have shown that *power napping for only six minutes is enough to significantly enhance memory.* Researchers at Harvard Medical School suggest that this memory enhancement occurs because the working memory has a chance to be sorted out and tidied up – information is taken from short-term stores to more durable long-term stores. This is possibly why you might remember more when you come out of your nap and also be able to take in more information as you have freed up space in your mental 'inbox'. So maybe the next time you are caught napping on the job you can quote the research!

Some sleep therapists advise against napping however, my experience has shown me that napping can not only help to alleviate the fatigue and other medical problems that can be caused by insomnia but also it can actually help to rebuild that vital connection with your sleep if it has become broken.

So what do I actually mean by 'napping' and can anyone nap? Many of my sleep-deprived patients and clients actually say 'I can't nap. I can never fall asleep during the day'.

There are different types of napping and each has its own value:

Replacement napping – these are naps that you take if you feel you have missed out on some of your sleep at

night and are feeling fatigued. I often recommend these
naps for athletes who are training heavily and to help
with injury recovery. *These naps typically last around 40-
50 mins but no more.* Any more time than this would take
you into the first stage of deep sleep and you will come
out of the nap feeling tired and groggy – this is called
sleep inertia. Napping for too long might also reduce
your need for sleep at night which could add to your
sleep problems.

Prophylactic napping – these are naps taken in advance of
sustained wakefulness. I recommend this type of napping
for my clients who work night shifts and can anticipate
that they are going to be missing out on sleep. These naps
last longer than replacement naps and can go on for as
long as the person is able to sleep.

Appetitive or power napping – these are naps that can be
taken even if you are not necessarily feeling fatigued. These
naps are also referred to as **ultra short naps** and are
typically 10–20min in duration. The most important thing
to understand about a power nap is that *it is not sleeping*. So
what is it? Here is my definition:

*A power nap is 10-20 minutes in which you will be aware of
thoughts, noises and sensations but at the same time will be in a
deep state of relaxation – not asleep but not awake.*

The benefits of such napping are many:

It is a great way of quickly lifting your energy without any
sleepiness afterwards.
Anyone can learn how to do it.
It is a great way of attuning the body to rest and then sleep at
the end of the day.

This last point is important. I have clients who have had terrible problems sleeping and for them, sleep has literally become the enemy. As a client said to me, 'I hate the thought of going to bed. As soon as I get into bed, my brain switches into overdrive and I just lie there becoming more and more anxious about not sleeping.' Nicola ran her own business and was a single parent with a 7-year old daughter. Her life was demanding and her days were busy with very little downtime. She agreed to try powernapping for 10 minutes in the afternoon before collecting her daughter from school. Sometimes she even did this in her car. After a few weeks of doing this Nicola's energy had lifted, she was noticeably calmer *and* her sleep had improved.

So now it's over to you. As before, read through the instructions thoroughly or pre-record them before attempting the technique.

5 Steps to power napping

STEP 1:

The first question you may have is 'when should I power nap?' The best time to power nap is during the day when you start to feel sleepy or your ability to concentrate on your task is reduced. You may have had the experience of this while driving for a long period of time or as many of us find, you have a lull or dip in your energy levels mid-afternoon around 3pm. This is the best time to take a power nap.

The first step is to get comfortable but not *too* comfortable. So avoid getting into bed and pulling the duvet up to your neck. You can use this technique just about anywhere where you can fully relax: a couch, a car, even the floor – the key is to find somewhere that you can mentally and physically relax without worrying about being disturbed.

Don't forget to switch off your phone. You might want to think about sound and lighting levels. I now power nap on noisy trains but when you first start using this technique you may want to experiment with creating an optimal environment for your power nap. This might involve using some relaxing aromatherapy oils in a burner or, if you have had a particularly busy day and your mind is racing, it might be helpful to have some sort of noise in the background that you can focus on to and ignore at the same time. White noise can be particularly effective for this. If you choose music, choose something relaxing and avoid anything with too much of a beat. You can experiment by dimming the light but avoid complete darkness.

STEP 2

Set an alarm for 10–20 mins or ask someone to let you know when this time has passed.

STEP 3

Close your eyes and become aware of your breathing. Move into the **NODS** sequence – Notice your breath, Open it up, Deepen your breathing, Slow down your breathing. You will be aware of external sounds, internal sensations and thoughts but keep focusing on your breathing and don't try to block anything out.

STEP 4

While focusing on your breathing, mentally whisper the word IIIIIIN as you breathe in and OOOOOOOUT as you breathe out. Feel yourself sinking deeper and deeper into relaxation with every breath you take. Focus on how your nostrils feel as the air moves in and out, or how the air feels when it hits the back of your throat.

STEP 5

When the alarm goes, rouse yourself gently from your nap. Open your eyes slowly and start to move your fingers and toes. After a minute or two you should be fully conscious, more relaxed and at the same time mentally and physically energised. If you can, take a short walk – 2 or 3 minutes will do or move around and do some gentle stretches.

You've done it! You have power napped! It really is as simple as that.

VARIATIONS

You can really optimise the results of your power nap by using your own relaxing words or mantra while you nap. For example, some people use the word 'calm' or 'peace'. Some people also use visualisation during their nap – this is a trick that many top athletes use to enhance their performance. You can start off by visualising the beach scene and the waves as you learnt in the Surfing the Breath tool. The sky really is the limit and the more you use this wonderful tool, the more creative you can be.

For even more energy and deeper relaxation, try combining this tool with the Pre-Sleep Yoga or the Legs up the Wall routines.

Caffeine napping – I know I have come down hard on caffeine but if you are really tired and need a big boost to your concentration, then some people find that combining caffeine with power napping can do the trick. The way to do it is to have a cup of coffee or tea beforehand and then go for your power nap. The caffeine doesn't stop you napping but kicks in after the nap. I personally find that using some good quality energising aromatherapy oils (for example, eucalyptus, menthol or citrus oils) can also have the same energising effect. Just put a few drops of the oils into a cup of hot water before you settle down for your nap and let the scents diffuse into the room while you nap.

What to expect from napping

Initially you may feel as if nothing really happened during your power nap or that all you did was to become aware of your thoughts. Stick with it and you will begin to notice that your thoughts slow down and become somewhat dream-like. This is when you know that you are truly relaxing and your mind is refreshing itself.

You may notice that after your power nap you feel more energised and that your eyes feel refreshed. This is exactly what you are looking for.

You might feel more tired after the power nap. Some of my more 'wired' clients experience this because they actually are very tired and this highlights their fatigue level. This effect usually diminishes with time and as you get used to power napping. The important thing is to use an alarm to rouse you and *avoid over-napping, as this really will make you tired and may reduce your need for sleep at night.*

Eventually you will find that you won't need to use an alarm as you become more proficient at using this technique and the brain's own innate sense of timing does the work for you.

The important thing is to experiment and find what really works for you. Throughout the writing of this book I have used power napping whenever I can to keep my energy, focus and concentration levels high. When I power nap in my office, I do so resting on a beanbag, in a room with the lighting low but not completely dark. I put a few drops of some balancing aromatherapy oils into a cup of hot water. I put my white noise machine on the 'rainfall' setting and set the timer for 15 minutes. I come out of my power nap when the machine stops and then I take a few minutes to gently bring myself back into full consciousness. I am then ready to resume writing with my batteries fully charged again.

REMEMBER:

- The OBT forms the basis for all of these power tools. Make sure that you are familiar with this technique before moving on to the advanced variations.
- Any of these tools can be used if you are having difficulties getting to sleep, staying asleep or if your mind is buzzing.
- Don't forget to combine all of these tools with the 'not checking the time' tool.
- For the best results, experiment and practice regularly.
- Combine with tools from other compartments for maximum benefit.

CHAPTER 10

Power Tools (III) – Mind Power

These tools will not only refine and deepen your sleep, but will also help you to achieve the inner feelings of safety and peace that are so vital to our wellbeing. I have described many times how the noisiness of thoughts and thinking can disrupt your sleep. Whereas the power tools I have described thus far have employed breathing and body work to help you relax and sleep, the tools in this section of the toolkit employ the power of the mind to help you achieve brilliant sleep. The Mind Power tools work on several levels:

1. They help you to become **aware** of unhelpful thoughts that can stop you sleeping.
2. They help you to step back and **observe** your thoughts rather than becoming overwhelmed by them.
3. They help you to **replace** unhelpful thoughts and patterns of thinking with more helpful ones.
4. They help you to **slow down** racing thoughts.

5. They help you to create an **inner core of peace and safety**.

I hope that by gaining a greater understanding of your thinking process you can gain greater control over your sleep.

Thinking thinking thinking . . .

We are what we think.
All that we are arises with our thoughts.
With our thoughts we make our world.

                                                    – The Buddha

No one really knows exactly how many thoughts we think in a day but it is estimated to be in the region of tens of thousands! According to some theories, human beings made the leap from stone tools to moonwalk by developing our patterns of thinking and, specifically, by evolving our ability to process complex information and memories. So clearly, thinking is a sophisticated process that sets us apart from less-evolved species. But there is a big difference between thinking consciously and constructively and using your intellect to generate helpful thoughts, and thoughts that seem to bubble up of their own accord whether you want them to or not. Particularly, when they become obsessive, ruminative and worrying.

Why is it that just when everything is quiet the volume of your thoughts seems to increase? Well actually you've been thinking all along but you have probably only become aware of it when you stop and try to get to sleep. That 'noise' has probably been in your head all along but you've effectively blocked it out with other distractions and the stuff of your daily life. Many people actually hate silence and will do anything to avoid it — they engage in excessive busyness, distract themselves

with hours of mind numbing television, over-indulge in alcohol or drugs. Anything to block out the sound of their own
internal noise. For many of my patients and clients this is what
creates their version of Tired but Wired – the relentless noise of
the day and the deafening 'silence' when they stop and become
aware of their thoughts.

Different types of thoughts can sabotage your sleep. First of
all, there are random thoughts containing fragments of the day
or, as one of my clients recently put it, 'it just feels as if I am
downloading my entire day'. Then there are the *worrying* or
what if thoughts. These usually involve thinking about what
might happen and catastrophising. And then they go around
and around gathering pace and become *racing* or *circling*
thoughts. Our attention yoyos back and forth between the past
and a make-believe scary future. In fact we are anywhere but in
the present. Buddhists describe the mind, when it is in this
state, as the *Monkey* Mind, as it is at its most mischievous and
seemingly, uncontrollable.

Thoughts can disrupt your sleep in three ways:

1. They stop you falling asleep
2. They stop you staying asleep – waking you in the early
   hours of the morning. Usually these thoughts are of the
   ruminative, worrying nature and are the ones that not
   only seem far worse at night but will stop you getting
   back to sleep
3. They 'crowd' into your sleep giving you the noisy, non-
   restorative sleep I have already described so many times.
   This is the kind of sleep that makes you feel as if you
   haven't slept at all.

I hope that in reading this you are experiencing some degree of
reassurance and maybe even relief; you are not alone in having

troublesome thoughts that get in the way of your sleep! So let's now look at how you can stop this happening.

Many of the techniques you have learnt about so far – and hopefully, started practising – will actually help to slow down this thinking process by allowing you greater control over your ability to relax and sleep. For example, cutting back on caffeine will dramatically smooth out the noise. Practising the breathing and relaxation techniques in the previous power tools sections will help to alleviate worrying and fear by helping you to feel safe about being in the present, as well as helping to create that internal chemistry that is essential for good sleep. What I will now share with you are the tools that work directly on your thinking process, smooth out the noise and help to create deep, peaceful sleep. I am going to start with some very simple techniques and then move toward the ones that work on a deeper level.

Mind Power 1: Time to worry

My life has been filled with terrible misfortune, most of which has never happened.

– Michel de Montaigne

This is the tool that will help you deal with all of those worries and anxieties that seem to surface *just* when you are trying to get to sleep. For all its simplicity, it is a gem. This is about creating some time and space to allow your anxieties and worries to have some free rein *outside of your sleep*. In other words, give yourself time to worry but not when you are sleeping. Intrusive worries and thoughts often get in the way of sleep when they are not being dealt with during the day and are being held back or repressed. I'm sure that there are times when you have said to yourself 'I just don't want to think about *that* right now.' The problem arises when *that* comes back to haunt you at 3am when all is quiet and you have all the time in the world to worry and fret.

So if your worries are stopping you from sleeping, get a piece of paper and a pen and list *everything* that is worrying you. Don't hold back. Really go for it. Sometimes my clients are afraid that by doing this they will become overwhelmed, but it is better to be overwhelmed by a black and white list in front of you than having all of the worries swirling around in your head in the early hours.

You might want to add to your list another column entitled 'The Worst Possible Scenario'. So what is the worst thing that could happen in this situation? What is the likelihood of it happening? And could you deal with it if it did happen?

Another way of using this tool would be to allow your 'creative' brain to get involved in helping you deal with your problems by creating a worry 'mind map' and rather than writing a list you get a large sheet of paper (whatever colour you fancy) and then, in separate areas on the paper, write down the main 'worry' categories. You may even choose to use sketches or images instead of words. Then for each category, write or sketch anything related to that worry or, alternatively, try to come up with as many solutions for each category as possible. For more on mind mapping I would direct you to Tony Buzan's *The Mindmap Book*.

Working with your worries and anxieties in this way allows them the space to be confronted and maybe even solved. You are using the combined power of your intellect and creativity to help you evaluate the situation, weigh up the options and help you make some discerning choices. The problem with worrying during your 'sleep time' is that when we sleep we become childlike, and our imagination takes off (you will learn more about this in the next chapter when we look at dreaming). This childlike state is great for creativity but it can sometimes work against us and problems can become ghoulish and magnified at night, when during the day they seem much more manageable.

Mind Power 2: The Perfect Bedtime Story

These next tools work on many levels – they help you to feel calm and relaxed but most importantly, and I have witnessed this many times, they help to build that 'inner core of safety' that I have already referred to so many times.

As you have learnt, there is a strong link between safety and your ability to sleep. It is a primitive and vital connection. But how do you create this connection? These tools will help to strengthen this safety connection by putting a good 'story' into your head before you go to sleep. In other words, they make it safe to sleep.

Just as I invited you earlier on when you looked at your wind down rituals to think about what you *do* before going to bed, I want you to think about what you *think* before you go to bed. Are your thoughts peaceful, secure or loving or are they frightening, worrying or even panicky? For many of my patients and clients what they do before they go to bed (non-relaxing TV, checking share prices, working on their lap top) fuels these anxious thoughts and stops them getting to sleep. I encourage them to replace these thoughts with one of my perfect bedtime stories.

THE OPTIMISM EXERCISE

This first variation on the perfect bedtime story is currently one of my favourite exercises; there is so much uncertainty in the world at the moment and it is so easy to get caught up in a whirlwind of pessimism and fear. This 'collective' anxiety is what stops many of my clients from sleeping.

There are many well-validated scientific studies showing a strong link between optimism and good health. Of particular note is the work of Martin Seligman, the psychologist and author of *Learned Optimism*. Seligman's work and research has very convincingly shown that optimists recover faster from setbacks and are able to act again sooner because of the way they explain the failure to themselves. His work and the work of other scientists has also shown that thinking positively can slow down or even reverse the progression of terminal illnesses such as cancer. But can you learn how to become more optimistic? Well, there is no doubt that you can and if this is something you would like to do then a good place to start would be to take a look at his book.

However, most importantly, given that you are reading this to get better sleep, I have noticed that 'optimism' tools can actually be used to create brilliant sleep. In the past year or so I have been teaching this simple Optimism Exercise to virtually every group I work with and the results have always been the same – the general feeling and energy of the group visibly lifts and people actually start smiling.

Let's do an exercise right now. I want you to put the book down and make sure that you have to hand a clock or watch with a second hand.

THE SIXTY SECOND OPTIMISM EXERCISE

60 seconds . . .

I now want you to give yourself 60 seconds (and no more) to come up with a mental or written list of ten positive things that have happened in your day from waking up this morning to now.

Could you do it? If you came up with seven or more – well done! If you came up with less than five, you really need to work on this. You may have noticed that some of the things you came up with were tiny – a nice cup of tea, a smile from someone, getting a seat on the train. It really doesn't matter what you come up with as long as you are able to recognise a positive element in it. I once had a patient who attended my hospital group for several weeks before he was able to come up with a single positive thing. He was a recovering alcoholic and had lost everything to his addiction – his business, his family, his money – and he was very depressed. I knew that he had turned the corner when he was able to identify one good thing in his day – the fact that he had woken up and was glad to be alive. Not surprisingly, this coincided with him starting to sleep well.

And now, applying this exercise to get good sleep . . . When you are in bed at night, allow yourself to relax and you might even practise the optimal breathing technique to help you do so. Now close your eyes, bring your attention inwards and cast your mind over the day's events in reverse (so you might see yourself reversing out of bed, going into the bathroom, cleaning your teeth etc). As you reverse through your day, try to think of every positive thing that has happened in your day – no matter how small or seemingly minor. If you lose concentration or start to think about something else, gently guide yourself to the point you drifted off at. My clients who use this tool regularly say that they not only fall asleep more easily, but they are more likely to stay asleep (or, at least, don't recall waking during the night) and wake up with more energy.

THE GRATITUDE EXERCISES

These exercises are subtle variations on the optimism exercise but with the vital element of *giving thanks*. Gratitude is a fundamental component of most spiritual paths, and a growing body of research in the field of positive psychology suggests that, like optimism, it has significant health benefits including better sleep. Dr Robert Emmons, a psychologist at the University of California, conducted a series of studies in 2003 in which he found that people who kept weekly written records of gratitude not only slept longer but experienced sleep that was deeper and more restorative. So here's how you can get started on your own gratitude practice . . .

Exercise 1: The way to do this is to again reverse through your day, acknowledge each positive thing that has happened to you and then give thanks for it. This might sound odd — whom do you thank for a nice cup of tea? This might depend on your religious beliefs and you might thank God or Allah, the Buddha or your Higher Self. If you have no such beliefs, it doesn't matter. Just acknowledging that you have something to be grateful for may produce that softening of attitude and letting go that is so essential for peaceful sleep.

Exercise 2: Another way of using the power of gratitude to improve your sleep is to keep a gratitude diary for 30 days. The way to do this is quite simple. Just take a pen and a piece of paper and write down all of the things that have happened in your day for which you can be grateful. I would encourage you to get everything down from getting to work in time to receiving a bonus at work. The best time to do this exercise is as a part of your wind down routine and you can even do it sitting comfortably in bed. If you are feeling anxious and overwhelmed by your day, you can even combine this exercise with the Tme to Worry tool – write out a list of all of your worries and when you have done this as completely as you can then turn to your gratitude diary and just start writing. My clients who practice the exercise regularly are often amazed by not only how long the list is but also how more good things just seem to keep coming their way afterwards.

Exercise 3: A beautiful, and powerful version of the gratitude exercise is one that has been adapted from ancient Buddhist philosophy by my friend and transformational life coach Gosia Gorna. Gosia works with cancer patients and uses this specific exercise with them with amazing results. Here's how you do it:

Get comfortable in bed, relax and breathe deeply from your belly. Feel yourself softening and letting go with each breath.

Bring to mind the thought or image of someone who is in your life that you are immensely grateful to. It may be someone in your immediate family or a friend. Hold their image in your mind and then bring it down into your heart. Allow yourself to feel what you feel when you think about them. Breathe into those feelings for a few minutes.

Now bring to your mind something that is going to be happening in your life for which you are grateful. It might be something very small but you are glad that it is going to be happening. You are looking forward to it.

Again, bring this into your heart and allow yourself to feel the feelings that arise when you do so.

Finally, and this is the most important part of the exercise, bring to your mind something about yourself that you are grateful for. Some habit or trait – no matter how small – but it is something that you are grateful for and that serves you well. As before, bring it into your heart, breathe deeply and feel how this makes you feel.

This lovely exercise, when used by Gosia with her patients, is normally practised in a daily meditation. However, I have found that it is particularly powerful when practised before sleep and over time can help you to cultivate not only optimism and gratitude but also the self-acceptance and softness that is essential for peaceful sleep.

YOUR OWN PERFECT BEDTIME STORY

Now this is an unusual tool as it is one that *you create for yourself*. But don't worry, I am going to show you exactly how to do this.

The aim is to create a bedtime story that is *just right for you* and has the perfect ingredients to help you feel relaxed, safe and able to let go and sleep. To help you find these ingredients, you just need to think about something you really enjoy doing, run through it in your mind like a film and slooooow it right down. It really is that simple. To illustrate what I mean, I am going to share with you the perfect bedtime stories of some of my clients.

The Italian Feast – in this story my client, who loves cooking sumptuous Italian food, imagines that she is in her kitchen getting together all of the ingredients to make her delicious pasta sauce. She gets the pan out of the cupboard, the knife and chopping board. She goes out into the garden to pick her fresh herbs. She slowly and carefully selects and picks each leaf, enjoying the colours and smells of the herb garden. She chops onions, hears them sizzle as they hit the hot oil in the pan, slowly chops the vibrant red tomatoes.

I am sure you are beginning to get the gist of this . . . The important thing is that your perfect story unravels in super slow motion with the greatest attention to detail as if it were really happening.

Cars and More Cars – this story comes from my husband who very rarely has problems sleeping (in fact, he's probably a Martini sleeper) and he loves cars. On the very rare occasion that he does have problems sleeping, he imagines that he has won a very large sum of money in the lottery. He uses the money to construct his garage of ultimate high performance cars. He then goes to each car, customising and adapting the specifications to his exact taste. Again, this is all done in slow motion.

Now this particular story is my idea of a nightmare, as I have no particular interest in cars. But I am sure you can appreciate the effect it might have on someone who is an automobile enthusiast.

The Perfect Home – another story comes from a wealthy client who loves decorating her beautiful home. In her perfect bedtime story, she moves slowly from one room to the next in her large house and designs the furniture, fittings, colours, and upholstery.

The First Kiss – Finally, this is one of my favourites and it came from one of my patients at the hospital, an attractive lady in her fifties. In her perfect bedtime story, she imagines going slowly back in time to all of her boyfriends and imagining the first kiss. She goes right back to the beginning starting with her first boyfriend. When she shared this with the group, everyone dissolved into fits of giggles and another patient commented that she 'couldn't think of anything worse!' But the point is, it really needs to be *your* story and yours only.

So what would be your perfect bedtime story? Can you conjure up an image of something that you love doing, that isn't too stimulating and can make you feel relaxed, peaceful and even sleepy?

Mind Power 3: Now I lay me down to sleep . . .

This tool is another of my personal favourites and one that works particularly well with children. It brings together beautifully the powerful ingredients of optimism and gratitude and can be considered to be the ultimate form of prayer for signing the day off. To practise this exercise all you do is before you go off to sleep ask yourself two questions:

What went well in my day today? No matter how tough your day has been or how many difficulties you have had to face, dig deep and try to come up with at least one or two things.

And now for your second question.

What am I looking forward to tomorrow? Again, dig deep if you have to. Try to come up with something, no matter how small it may seem. I use this technique particularly when I'm feeling nervous about something happening the next day – a big presentation for example. I really work on focusing on the tiny things that are within my control that I can look forward to. For example, getting into my car and enjoying listening to a particular piece of music specially chosen for the journey, or focusing on particular aspects of the presentation that I know I do well.

Invariably, when I use this technique, I not only fall asleep effortlessly but I wake up with energy and looking forward to the day ahead. We all need a reason to get out of bed in the morning, a sense of *purpose*. When we pay attention to our need for purpose, amazing things can happen to our sleep.

Mind Power 4: Meditation

I have never missed a meditation in thirty-three years. I meditate once in the morning and again in the afternoon, for about twenty minutes each time. Then I go about the business of my day. And I find that the joy of doing increases. Intuition increases. The pleasure of life grows. And negativity recedes.

> – 'Catching the Big Fish' David Lynch, film director

I consider this to be the *ultimate power tool for honing and creating brilliant sleep*. Meditation works by allowing the mind to settle down and de-excite. Practised regularly it helps you become aware of unhelpful thoughts, detach yourself from them, slow them down, thus reducing the internal noise and buzziness. Once we become aware that our thoughts are unhelpful and are able to observe them, rather than becoming immersed in and overwhelmed by them, then we can choose to do something about them or replace them with more helpful thoughts – such as the ones I have described previously in the perfect bedtime stories.

I had spent years using my sleep tools to optimise the quality of my own sleep but it was when I started meditating that I truly learnt the meaning of brilliant sleep. I have now been recommending meditation to my patients and clients for many years and have witnessed time and again the transformation it brings to their sleep, energy levels and wellbeing.

Meditation has been around for a long time – at least 5,000 years – but only really became popular in the Western world in the 1960s. Most meditation practices are based on ancient philosophy and religious practices, but can be adapted for use in today's modern world. In fact, I believe that this is where meditation can have its greatest benefits: not on a beautiful, mountaintop overlooking a perfectly still lake but in today's noisy, information-filled, driven world. What follows is not a detailed set of instructions on how to meditate – I believe it would be hard to learn how to meditate from a book. Furthermore, even after years of meditating, I still consider myself to be a novice. However, what I would like to share with you is an overview of how meditation can help you sleep better as well as offering you a few basics on how to establish your own meditation practice.

The word meditation is derived from two Latin words: meditari (to think, to dwell upon, to exercise the mind) and mederi (to heal). Its Sanskrit derivation 'medha' means wisdom. Many people mistakenly believe that it is a state of complete and total non-thinking – and this is what often causes them to abandon their practice. 'I find it impossible to meditate. I just can't stop thinking!' This is the most common statement I hear about meditation – people complaining of their inability to stop thinking. So, let me repeat what I said earlier, *meditation isn't about trying to create a state of non-thinking.* Meditation is about observing the thinking process, becoming aware of it, accepting and allowing it to happen while gently guiding and directing your focus to something else such as your breathing or a mantra. Most of all, meditation involves letting go, accepting what comes up in your mind, inviting softness and stillness into your being. In short, all of the vital ingredients for deep, nourishing sleep.

What happens when you first start meditating? Well, for a

number of people it may seem as if nothing happens. My personal experience of my first meditation was of feeling very peaceful for a few minutes and then a bubbling up of impatience – 'How long is this going to take? I've got so much to do!' In subsequent sessions, I became very aware of the noisiness of my thoughts, the silliness of my thoughts, the apparent randomness of my thoughts. But then over time I became more an observer of my thoughts, less inclined to get caught up in the stories, the worries and anxieties. I also began to notice the difference in the clarity of my thoughts during the day and then, most importantly, I noticed how much easier it was to fall asleep – even after a busy day – and how much more peaceful and restorative my sleep felt.

So why does meditation affect sleep in this way? There is a solid body of evidence from well-validated neurophysiological studies showing that meditation significantly improves sleep quality because of the impact on breathing and the nervous system. Meditation also seems to act directly on the brain actually 'sculpting' the brain and changing its very structure and wiring. Most significantly, when practised regularly meditation seems to develop within you that inner core of peace and safety that is so vital for brilliant sleep.

I hope you are now starting to become interested in the idea of starting your own practice. So how do you do this? First of all I would recommend finding a good meditation course. There are so many different types of meditation and, like I once did you may find it a little bewildering when thinking about where to start. Please have a look at the Further Resources section at the back of the book and you will find some information on recommended reading and meditation workshops.

However, to start with, you might want to experiment with creating your own meditation practice using some of the techniques I have already described to you. Here's how you could do it:

THE 5 MINUTE MEDITATION

Find a quiet space where you will be undisturbed for 5 minutes. Sit down and close your eyes. It is best if you can practice without any music. Bring your attention to your breathing and just watch the rise and fall of your breath. You will become aware of thoughts drifting through your mind but just keep coming back to your breath.

It is important not to try to block your thoughts out but rather to simply observe them without becoming caught up and involved in them. Let them come and pass. If one thought is dominating your mind just watch it and then notice how the next thought comes and supersedes the current thought. Keep doing this for a few minutes. Just watching your thoughts rise up like bubbles and then pass. Each time you find yourself getting involved in a thought, just gently detach yourself from it and watch it. Wait for the next thought to 'bubble up' again.

If it helps you to focus more easily, try mentally and softly whispering the word IN as you breathe in and OUT as you breathe out. Alternatively, you might want to choose your own word such as CALM or PEACE. In many meditation practices you are actually given your own personal mantra to focus on. Continue following your breathing or repeating your word for the entire 5 minutes. If during this time you need to open your eyes to check the time, do so and then close your eyes and resume your meditation. At the end of the 5 minutes, keep your eyes closed and allow yourself a minute or two to gently bring yourself to full consciousness with your eyes open. When you have finished your meditation avoid rushing full tilt back into your day, but try to maintain the state of relaxation as you go about your day.

WHAT TO EXPECT

What was your experience of doing this exercise?

Some of my clients find this exercise quite maddening when they first start using it. 'Sitting here listening to the rubbish in my head is *so* annoying!' said Matthew, a 17yr old school boy. However, after a fortnight of regular practice, Matthew noticed that he fell asleep more easily and that his sleep felt so much more peaceful. He was also amazed to find that he was able to think much more clearly during the day and felt less 'hyper'.

If you have never done anything like this before it might have seemed very strange – maybe even a waste of time. Part of the strangeness of this exercise may lie in the fact that you are seemingly focusing on nothing apart from the bubbling up of your thoughts. It may have seemed as if your mind was full of thoughts and that you were thinking too much. But remember, *you* are not thinking about anything; thoughts are just passing. In this way, by stepping back from and observing your thoughts, no thought can take root and your mind will begin to unload information faster.

The important thing is to stick with the technique even if it initially feels as if you are doing nothing. Trust me, this can really make a difference.

YOUR MEDITATION PRACTICE

To build this into a meditation practice that will truly optimise the quality of your sleep, you really do need to practice regularly and there is no way around this. I have emphasised the need for regular practice with all of the tools I have described in the Sleep Toolkit but this is *especially* the case for meditation – *regular practice is what will get you results.* So how do you create a regular practice? Well, you simply set aside time every day to meditate. You might choose to do this every morning as soon as you wake up or every evening when you start to wind down. You may choose to meditate twice a day – once in the morning and once in the evening. Use the following guidelines to create your own meditation practice:

1. Create an intention to meditate *every* day no matter what happens – remember this is going to get you the brilliant sleep you really want. You have got to make it *imperative* – in the same way as you make it imperative to put your clothes on before leaving your house. Link it to your *vision* for your sleep. Remember what you are trying to achieve and hold this intention to help keep you on track.

2. Decide roughly what sort of time(s) you will aim to meditate. For example, I meditate as soon as I wake up and then again at some point between 4 and 7pm.

3. Don't meditate more than twice per day.

4. Decide what form of meditation you will use. Will you focus on your breath or use a word or mantra?

5. Decide how long you will meditate for – you might want to start with 5 minutes every morning for the first fortnight and then work up to doing 20 minutes every morning. Always come out of your meditation slowly.

6. Don't allow yourself to lapse from the habit – 1 or 2 days of not meditating will set you back and make it more difficult to establish a habit.

7. Be flexible in your attitude – think of your meditation practice as highly 'portable'. I now meditate in cars, on planes and trains, or even in my client's offices if I need to. I have now become very used to meditating in noisy surroundings.

8. Plan ahead wherever possible. For example, if you know you've got an evening engagement to go to, meditate before you go out.
9. Don't meditate after drinking alcohol.
10. Avoid meditating *immediately* before you get into bed. This can actually energise you and you may find it harder to get to sleep!

The value of all of the Mind Power Tools you have just learnt about lies in the fact that they help you to build separation between you and your thoughts. By getting them out of your head by writing them down or by just observing them, you detach from them and they lose their power over you. As one of my clients said to me, 'I now just say hello and goodbye to my 'anxiety thoughts' when they pop up and they have stopped controlling me.'

In the next section of the toolkit, we are going to stay with the theme of the mind and how it can influence your sleep by looking at the thoughts and images that can bubble up from your unconscious while you sleep – the fascinating process of *dreaming*.

REMEMBER:
- Gaining control over your thoughts and thinking processes is key to creating brilliant sleep.
- Create some time to address your worries and anxieties outside of your sleep. Set aside some time and write a list of all of the things that are worrying you.
- Replace unhelpful thoughts with a Perfect Bedtime Story.
- Use the power of Optimism or Gratitude to help you get to sleep, or create your own Perfect Bedtime Story.

- For peaceful sleep and more energy when you wake up give some thought to what went well in your day and make sure that you have something to look forward to the next day, no matter how small.
- Follow a regular meditation practice for your ultimate brilliant sleep.

CHAPTER 11

Power Tools (IV) – To Sleep Perchance to Dream

We never stop seeing, perhaps that is why we dream.

– Goethe

Do you remember dreaming last night? And if so, do you remember your dreams vividly or have they left in your mind just a vague and fleeting impression? By the way, I am not referring to the mundane, 'to-do list' dreaming where you wake up thinking 'Have I sent this email to my client?' or 'Have I paid my credit card bill?' Rather I am referring to the bizarre, strange and sometimes terrifying dreams that can wake us in the middle of the night or actually leave a bad taste in your mouth the next day.

I debated about whether or not to include a mini chapter on dreaming and Dream Tools and then, in a somewhat serendipitous fashion, just when I had decided not to, my own dreams seemed to become 'noisier' and more vivid. I also seemed to encounter more patients who wanted me to work with them specifically on their dreams. Maybe this is a version of the attentional bias I referred to earlier – was it because I was turning the spotlight on dreaming that I seemed to notice that there was more 'dream work' to do? Well whatever it was, something seemed to be guiding me to write a chapter on dreams.

Strictly speaking this chapter isn't really about how to interpret your dreams although by practising some of the tools you may start to get a better understanding of what your dreams are about. People tend to be as fascinated by their own dreams as they are bored rigid by everyone else's and I must confess that I occasionally get a sinking feeling when someone in one of my groups decides to spend 15 minutes describing the convoluted and ridiculous details of the dream they had the previous night. Don't get me wrong – sometimes I do find them fascinating especially when they come from my five-year-old daughter – but I am *not* an expert in dream interpretation and I am definitely not the one to talk to if you have recurring dreams about being Dorothy in the Wizard of Oz! For a fascinating insight into dreams and how to interpret them, I would point you in the direction of Robin Royston's excellent *The Hidden Power of Dreams*.

Now that I've cleared that up, what is this section about? Some of the people I work with, particularly the patients at the hospital, complain of disturbing dreams. For some, it might have been the disturbing dreams that actually played a big part in their problems with drugs or alcohol – in other words, their dreams had become so disturbing that they were desperately trying to repress or sedate them. For my clients in the 'well' world their dreams may not be as 'pathological' but may still have a disturbing element that stops them sleeping peacefully.

What follows are some practical ways of 'befriending' your dreams rather than running away from them. Some ways of understanding them and maybe even tapping into their hidden power. I believe that dreams can have a great ability to enhance your creativity and solve your problems as well as an amazing power to heal. I view the dreamwork that I do with my patients as vital to their recovery.

Remembering your dreams

On average, we have about six spells of dreaming throughout the night. We all dream but some of us remember our dreams much more readily than others. You may recall that most dreams occur during REM sleep or more precisely, during the hypnagogic trance state. To remind you, the latter is the stage of REM sleep that you experience just as you are emerging from or drifting into sleep. Sometimes you may experience this just before your alarm clock goes off and jolts you into consciousness and so these images and dreams might be the ones that leave the most vivid impression in your memory. These dreams are actually called **hypnopompic hallucinations** and although it may feel as if you have been having them all night, they may have only popped up in the moments before you woke up.

During REM sleep, the body goes into a state of paralysis to stop us from acting out our dreams. The exception to this is when you experience **night terrors** and then have no recollection of your dreams, as this is most likely to occur during deep, unconscious sleep. But the dreamer may be left feeling tired and uneasy the next day. **Sleep talking, sleepwalking** and **teethgrinding** are also most likely to occur during deep sleep so the sufferer will have no recollection of their nocturnal antics. Another exception are the nightmares that occur with **post-traumatic stress disorder (PTSD)** in non-REM sleep. The evidence suggests that these are not strictly dreams but are rather more like flashbacks that intrude into your wakeful consciousness.

So we are more likely to remember the dreams that we have during REM sleep than the ones that we have in deep sleep. But why do some people remember their dreams more vividly than others? And why do some people appear not to remember their dreams at all? For some people their dreams are so vivid that it is as if they are consciously directing their dreams even as they are aware that they are dreaming them. These are the so-called **lucid dreams**.

There are a number of theories about dream recall but the one that makes the most sense to me and is most consistent with what I encounter in my work relates to Dr Eric Hartmann's fascinating work on *thick and thin boundaries*. According to his theory, these 'boundaries' are the gaps in the brain that allow communication between the right side of the brain (the side that dreams) and the left side of the brain (the side that analyses and remembers). So in order to have good dream recall, you need to have good communication between these two sides of the brain. According to Hartmann's research, people who score high on empathy, are creative, more emotional and sensitive in nature are more likely to be 'thin boundaried' and, therefore, have a higher dream recall. On the other hand, those who are more practical, down-to-earth and maybe even thick-skinned are more 'thick boundaried' and less likely to remember their dreams.

The role of bizarre dreams

I once worked with a client who had been suffering from chronic fatigue and depression for a number of years. When she came to see me she was making good progress, had stopped taking her antidepressant medication and was thinking about taking further education courses and picking up the threads of her career. However, the reason she had come to see me was that more recently her sleep had been disrupted by nightmare-like dreams to the extent that she had become fearful of going to sleep. I tried to reassure her that this is actually a normal part of the recovery process and something I see with many people who are recovering from chronic illnesses or addictions and coming off medication – their dreams can return with an alarming ferocity – and I try to encourage them to treat their dreams like a friendly counsellor or best friend who is trying to help them to make sense and come to terms with what has happened in their lives.

I believe that bizarre, symbolic dreams can carry messages from our unconscious. They are helping us to give voice to something that is deep-seated and emotional – maybe even traumatic. In *Out of the Dark* Linda Caine and Robin Royston tell the true and compelling story of how Caine uncovers the dark secrets of her traumatic childhood through her dreams. The story also recounts how she works with Royston, a clinical psychologist, to make sense of her dreams and recover her sanity.

Sometimes my vivid dreamers are not just the creative or thin-boundaried types but also the ones who tend to hold back from expressing themselves. I see them as the 'swan-types' – calm and serene on the surface but with all of the activity happening below. Along with vivid dreams, these individuals might also grind their teeth – the bruxism I described earlier.

Dreams as a source of creativity

You may recall reading in Part I about the creative and problem solving potential of dreaming in the stories of Einstein's dream about riding a beam of light and Kekulé's dream that helped him to deduce the ring-like structure of benzene. So too your dreams may provide important insights into your creativity and actually help you to solve your problems. I'm sure there are times when you have gone to bed with a problem in your mind and then woken up in the morning feeling better about it and maybe even having found a solution. So 'sleeping on it' can sometimes be a very good idea.

Many of my clients are very creative types – artists, musicians, actors and actresses and writers – and their dreams are often creative and sometimes disturbing, particularly if they aren't expressing their creativity. Stephen King, in his book *On Writing* describes the dream that gave birth to one of his most popular stories. He fell asleep during a plane trip to London and had a dream...

'. . . *about a popular writer . . . who fell into the clutches of a psychotic fan living on a farm somewhere out in the back of the beyond. The fan was a woman isolated by her growing paranoia.*'

King woke from his vivid dream and scribbled it down on an American Airlines cocktail napkin. On arrival in London, he and his wife stayed in a hotel but he found himself unable to sleep – he put it down to a combination of jet lag and 'what was on that airline cocktail napkin'. He got up and spent the night writing sixteen pages of the story that was eventually to become the bestselling novel *Misery*.

Do you know if you are creative? Some of the people I work with are actually very creative but they don't realise it. It is only when they begin working with their dreams that they discover the nature of their creativity and peaceful sleep returns.

Dreams as premonitions

On the night after I began writing this chapter, I retired to bed feeling pleasantly tired and drifted off to sleep effortlessly. That night I had a vivid and disturbing dream in which I was on a train on my way to a meeting. The train stopped at my station and I disembarked but as the train pulled out of the station, I realised that I had left on board the train my handbag with the memory stick containing all of the files for **Tired but Wired!** I felt sick with panic when I realised that this was the *only* copy I had of my book. I began chasing the train and somehow managed to get back on board by flying through an open window. I ran through the compartments but couldn't find my handbag no matter how hard I looked. I kept asking people if they had seen my bag but no one seemed to hear me or take any notice of me. Eventually, I woke from my dream with a start, feeling panic-stricken and then relieved when I realised that it was only a dream. But somehow the feeling of that dream lingered with me all day and I felt somewhat uneasy . . . The feeling lifted when, later that day, I sat at my computer and made backup copies of the Tired but Wired files.

It is very possible that it had been at the back of my mind for a while that I should copy the files – this is common sense after all. But, rather irresponsibly, I hadn't done this. My dream was a bit of a wake-up call and a premonition of what could happen if I didn't do what needed to be done.

Dreams that confront fears

I once worked with a Premiership goalkeeper who occasion-ally had a particular recurring dream the night before a big football game. In his dream, he is standing on full alert on the goal line about to defend a penalty kick. The stadium is hushed and tense with anticipation. The footballer takes the kick, the ball heads into the net, the goalkeeper dives to block the ball – and misses. When he recounted his dream, I asked him if the dream made him feel anxious about playing the next day. To my surprise he said 'Absolutely not! It's great when I have this dream because I know this *won't happen* when I play on the day'. For him, this dream was a way of helping him to face his unconscious fear so that it didn't consciously affect his performance.

Dreams that heal

Royston's *The Hidden Power of Dreams* gives many fascinating accounts of dreams that have predicted illness, disasters and events. He also describes dreams that come from beyond that are of a more spiritual nature – I have certainly heard about such dreams from my clients and patients and have had them myself, especially after the sudden death of my sister in 2002. Such dreams, when given the space to be aired and understood, can be a great source of comfort and reassurance.

What I would now like to share with you are some tools that I myself have been practising and recommending to my patients and clients for many years. I have seen the great benefits and healing that they can bring and I hope you will find them a useful addition to your own Sleep Toolkit.

Taking the first step . . .

As I have already mentioned, your dreams can be viewed as a message from your subconscious to give voice to something. What follows are some simple exercises in journaling to help you do this. Using these regularly you may find that you are more able to make sense of your dreams and maybe even receive the messages they carry. You may also find that your dreams become less ferocious and are less likely to taint your day.

Many people are afraid to start writing about their dreams either because they worry about 'opening a can of worms' or not being able to write. Regarding the first worry let me remind you that when you begin expressing the intensity of your dreams will become softer and kinder. I've not only experienced this personally but I have seen this happening with my clients time and again. However, if your dreams are very distressing I would advise you to do any writing with the support of a professional, qualified and empathetic therapist or counsellor.

And about not being able to write – get out of your own way! Or as Sean Connery the university professor in *Finding Forrester* says to his student in 'Stop thinking and write!'

Get yourself the perfect pen or pencil and the right notepad or paper and then just get ready to write. Before you start writing it might be helpful to consider the following suggestions:

1. Before you fall asleep tell yourself, 'I am looking forward to remembering my dreams when I wake up'.
2. If possible, try to write as soon as you wake up and avoid talking about your dream before you write. This way, your memory is uncluttered with the noise of the day or other people's interpretations and should still hold the most recent memories of your dreams.
3. Don't try to force it. Just relax and breathe and allow the images and memories to slowly bubble up to the surface. Sometimes, in my first meditation of the day, I actually return to my dream and my dream recall is then much stronger.
4. Avoid trying to force any immediate analysis or interpretation of your dream. Try to write down as much as you can about your dream and then come back to your record later. Interpretation and analysis engages another part of your brain and to remember your dream as fully as you can, you need to keep your 'dreaming brain' open and engaged.

Stream of consciousness dream journaling

In her book *The Artist's Way* Julia Cameron refers to this type of journaling as *the morning pages* in which you transfer your first thoughts of the day into a journal. According to Cameron's morning pages method you write, with absolute unwavering discipline, three pages every morning. However, to help you become better acquainted with your dreams, I simply recommend that you write about your dreams whenever you can although, as I've already mentioned, first thing in the morning is always best to capture the true essence of your dream.

There is no right or wrong about how you do this. You may not choose to do this every day, after all there are some nights when your dreams are not particularly vivid or memorable. You might not even do it first thing in the morning. When I rise early for work, I have no time to sit and write – I'm too busy eating, showering, looking after my daughter and beginning my day. But when I get on my train, I scribble furiously for the twenty-five minutes of my journey. I don't do this every day but I *especially* do it on the days when my dreams have been particularly 'vocal' the night before. I see this as an essential 'clearing' that needs to be done before I can work with my clients.

There may be times when you don't have a clear memory of your dreams but rather a vague impression or sense of uneasiness when you wake up. In such instances, it may be particularly helpful to simply write about *how you feel* without probing your memory too deeply. Just let your pen just glide over the paper and you may then begin to recall snippets of your dreams.

Another important point is to drop the perfectionism. *It doesn't have to be perfect*. Stop editing. Forget everything you were told at school about punctuation and grammar and just write. Five lines or five pages – it doesn't matter how much you write. Just write.

In case you're still not sure about how to go about writing about your dreams, here are a few questions just to get you started and deepen the process of inquiry into your dream:

What happened in my dream?
How was I feeling?
What else might have been happening?
Is this really how I was feeling?
Is this account as clear as I can make it?

Try to write in the **present tense** to bring you closer into your dream.

Chaos narrative dream journaling

In *Writing as a Way of Healing* Louise DeSalvo recommends the 'chaos narrative' as a way of writing if you are in a state of crisis and are unable to put the words together in the sort of coherent sequence I have described above. Many of my patients have found that writing in this way can be a useful way of navigating to calmer waters when they are woken suddenly from a distressing dream. As one client said recently 'It gets it out of my head and puts it somewhere where I can look at it. If I can look at it I am not living it.'

Hannah, a 21-year-old PhD student, wrote the following when she woke from a particularly vivid dream:

'Hot/ sweating/ panic/ out of control/ too many people/ no-one listening/ too much noise/ can't speak/ my throat constricted/ can't breathe/ red face/ can't remember/ out of control.'

Hannah suffered from panic attacks and hated the idea of speaking in public, something she had to do as part of her doctorate. Once Hannah started journaling this particular recurring dream using chaos narrative it was as if, to use her words 'the bubble burst' and presenting in public became a lot easier for her.

What to expect

As with all of the tools in the Toolkit, regular usage will get you the best results. Sometimes, my clients are slightly disappointed when they first start journaling. They might have expected to get great flashes of inspiration and blinding revelations. You may be lucky and find that you do. What is more likely to happen is any of the following:

- Your sleep becomes more peaceful
- You feel more peaceful
- You feel a greater sense of vitality and well being
- You slowly start to gain more insight into your own dream process and the messages that lie within your dreams
- You are less likely to be distressed by vivid dreams and they are less likely to taint your day

When words just won't do . . .

Painting is just another way of keeping a diary.

– Pablo Picasso

Sometimes it is difficult to put words to the feelings that arise from having had disturbing dreams. You are simply just left with a bad feeling. For some of my clients, it is not writing that helps them to befriend their dreams but giving space to their creativity whether through art, singing, dance, music, poetry or even knitting! It doesn't matter what it is but the important thing is to find your creativity outlet and use it.

Get it off your chest!

And now for a little bit of silliness . . . What follows is a lovely little exercise that really can help you to express in a way that stops your dreams butting in to your sleep and it works especially well for those of you who grind your teeth at night. Practised regularly, it really does work – especially with children.

This tool is to do with expressing through sound and it comes from a variation of the 'lion posture' in yoga. I would recommend that you familiarise yourself with the following instructions, put the book down and have a go right now . . .

LION POSTURE EXERCISE

Get comfortable – you can stand, sit or kneel. Straighten up and relax your shoulders and neck.

The jaw 'waggle' – loosen your jaw by gripping your chin gently between finger and thumb and then 'waggling' your jaw. Try letting some sound through at the same time. If you can warble perfectly your jaw is nice and loose! If you find that your jaw is really 'tight' then you really need to do the next part of this exercise.

Inhale deeply through your nose, exhale forcefully through your mouth making an AAAAAAH sound while opening your mouth wide. Hold this for a few seconds then close your mouth and repeat the exercise and this time stretch your tongue out and down. Try opening your mouth a little wider each time.

Repeat the jaw waggle. Is your jaw looser now?

How did you get on with this exercise? You may have felt a bit silly but is your jaw now nice and loose? Did you manage to get a good AAAAAH going? The AAAH sound is the first primitive sound of distress that a human being makes. Just think about what babies do if they are hungry, tired, bored or in some other way distressed. They simply AAAAH! There is great therapeutic value to be had by making the AAAAH sound. Sometimes our pain or distress goes beyond verbal articulation – it's just a feeling of frustration, irritation or anger that needs to be gotten rid of. In fact, I had this very feeling this morning when my printer kept jamming and I ended up making this very sound in the privacy of my office! I didn't want to talk or write about how I felt about my printer jamming but neither did I want to hold on to the frustration I was feeling.

I'm sure you've had days when you've felt like making this sound (and very loudly) but it might have been inappropriate or career limiting. So we learn as we get older how to 'put the lid on it', put a smile on our face and go about our day as if nothing has happened. Some people are better at doing this than others – in my experience they are often best teethgrinders.

The bottom line is that when you fail to express what you feel it will probably pop up somewhere else – maybe in your dreams or in your clenched jaw. The important thing is to drop all self-consciousness and just use this tool regularly. The best time to do it is before you go to bed and just before you clean your teeth. You may well end up with more peaceful sleep as well as beautifully toned facial muscles!

DON'T FORGET THE BASICS...

To get the most out of these Dream Tools don't forget to keep using the Nuts and Bolts and Basic sleep tools. Allow me to illustrate my point . . .

I recently worked with Annie a patient who had suffered an extremely traumatic event a few years ago. Since then, she had been experiencing terrifying and recurring dreams in which she would wake up in a cold sweat, panicking, heart racing and then find herself unable to get back to sleep. Annie was having intense therapy with a psychologist but her dreams were still vivid and distressing. During our session she revealed that her caffeine intake was extremely high – more than ten cups of tea in a day – and her nutritional patterns were also very poor. I went back to some 'basics' with Annie, addressing her nutrition and getting her to cut back drastically on her caffeine intake. The result? Within a few days the intensity of her dreams had lessened. Although these measures did not solve all of her problems, they went a long way towards alleviating the distress that she was experiencing from her dreams.

With the final addition of these tools, I can now close the Sleep Toolkit and hand it over to you. You now have the complete set at your disposal and I hope you will enjoy putting together your own set of sleep tools and using them to create your brilliant sleep. But before you do so, I invite you to turn the page and read another two final stories. I hope you will find the first one very inspiring. The other story, my own, is less so and proves that sometimes even the experts don't get it right.

REMEMBER:

- We all dream whether we remember our dreams or not
- Your dreams may be a source of healing or creativity
- Our dreams could become louder and distressing if we don't allow them the space to be expressed

- Use journaling or a creative hobby to express the hidden power of your dreams
- Don't forget to use the Nuts and Bolts and Basic Tools to minimise the noisiness of your sleep

CHAPTER 12

Putting it all Together

This is probably going to sound a little clichéd but writing this book has been a journey. I've learnt more about the process of sleep, deepened my work with my clients and at the same time, learnt to sleep *even* better myself. I hope that you too have benefited from taking the time to read it and are already experiencing the joy of sleeping better and having more energy.

And now for one final story . . . Perhaps not as inspiring as some of the stories I've shared with you so far but it comes with a fair dollop of irony and a slight hint of the confessional about it . . . this is the story of how I've slept in the past two weeks.

Right at the beginning you learnt that I had once had my own fair share of sleep problems but that I now sleep brilliantly. Or at least most of the time I do. Recently my sleep has been abysmal! Getting to sleep has been no problem at all but my sleep has been noisy with vivid dreams – in short, somewhat Tired but Wired! I haven't slept this badly for years.

A wise person once said 'You teach what you need to learn'

and this has certainly been the case in terms of my relationship with sleep. Consequently I've had to go back to the Basics (and the Nuts and Bolts) to work out exactly what is going on with my sleep. To my surprise (and amusement), I've discovered that my own Sleep Toolkit is somewhat in a state of disarray. So based on my current experience of getting somewhat less than brilliant sleep, and in the interest of closing on a somewhat lighter note, I've compiled my top ten tips for getting Tired but Wired sleep:

1. Work at your computer until late into the night and then skip your wind down routine;
2. Consume a fair amount of chocolate or cake while doing so;
3. Read the 'Can't Put it Down' novel you had been saving for your holiday just before going off to sleep;
4. In the interest of saving time, skip the power breakfast (porridge with nuts and seeds) and go for sugar laden cereal with a strong cup of tea;
5. Pour yourself countless glasses of water which you never drink;
6. Avoid the fruit bowl and head for the biscuit tin when you get that mid-morning lull;
7. Grab a cup of coffee to wash it down;
8. Cut corners in your meditation – ten minutes will have to do;
9. Cut back on exercise and movement (you are writing a book after all);
10. Blame your poor sleep on being a troubled creative and having poor 'sleep genetics' thereby absolving yourself of any responsibility for doing anything about it.

Yes I know that I should know better but as I said a while ago, 'Knowledge is not wisdom,' and of late I have certainly been unwise about my sleep. I am a Sensitive sleeper and probably always will be so it's time to return to the Toolkit and start putting things back in order.

So it's over to you now. I hope that you now understand a great deal about your unique relationship with sleep. Most of all I hope that you are feeling motivated and even excited about the prospect of doing what needs to be done to take control of it. Remember I talked about the ARC of change – Awareness – Responsibility – Choices? Are you now ready to take responsibility for your sleep? Are you ready to make the choices that will enable you to sleep brilliantly?

Creating Sustainable Change

Don't forget, you're in this for the long haul and I want to be there with you too helping you to create the change that will last. There may be bumps in the road – times when it feels as if you really aren't making progress at all. Stick with it. Treat your sleep like the British Weather and be prepared for the occasional unexpected storm. Then let go of it and allow your sleep to readjust itself. Remind yourself of the vision you hold for your sleep to stop yourself relapsing. Keep reminding yourself that this isn't just about your sleep – pay attention to all of those other vital aspects of your energy and make the commitment to give them your attention too.

As Mahatma Gandhi once said, 'There is more to life than its increasing speed.' Indeed there *is* more to life than the feverish activity that we assume is our natural state. We need more time to cease *doing* and simply *be*. Time to rest, imagine, create, dream and sleep. When we do this we withdraw from the noisy outer world to be with ourselves, unburdened by the stresses and strains of daily life. As a result, we are more in balance and at ease, physically, mentally, emotionally and spiritually.

I used to think of my sleep as my curse and I now know that it is my gift and for that reason I must never take it for granted. I hope that you will keep this book with you as your constant bedside companion as a reminder to keep you on the path of deep, nourishing and healing sleep. **Most of all, I wish you brilliant sleep and the energy to live the kind of life you truly want to live.**

Part Three

TAKING ACTION

The final part of this book comprises two brief chapters. Chapter 13 is an in-depth case study illustrating the Sleep Toolkit in action. Chapter 14 is a collection of some of the questions I am frequently asked about sleep problems, and a helpful index of the sleep toolkit for easy reference.

Karen B. Learns How to Sleep Brilliantly

I want to share one last story with you. Karen B. came to see me just at the point when I was nearing completion of the manuscript. Initially I thought twice about taking on more work when I needed to keep my head down and focus on writing. But despite the challenge she presented, working with her proved to be such a success and so, with her permission, I decided to share her story with you. I do this in the hope that it will inspire you to keep going in your quest for good sleep and greater vitality and to encourage you to believe that it *really* is possible for you to sleep brilliantly even if you have suffered a lifelong history of insomnia.

Karen's Story

Karen came to see me not as a patient or client but as a colleague who had heard about my work with sleep and energy and, as a dedicated doctor, wanted to know if there was anything she herself could do to help her patients.

When I first met Karen I was struck by an apparent contradiction – while she was a very buzzy, high-energy type at the same time I could sense within her a deep underlying fatigue. Sitting on the edge of her seat, she spoke very quickly and animatedly but at the same time there was what I can only describe as a 'greyness' to her energy that I couldn't quite fathom.

I asked her, 'How do you sleep Karen?' To which she replied half-jokingly 'don't even go there! My sleep is awful and always has been. My whole family are like this and I don't think there's much I can do about it really.' I probed deeper, 'How do you feel? What are your energy levels like?' Karen immediately answered 'Awful! Some of the time I am driven by something that feels very buzzy and I just have to keep going but the rest of the time I'm exhausted'.

And then Karen had a brainwave, 'Do you think you could help me to have more energy? You probably can't do anything about my sleep problems because they are so long-standing, and probably genetic anyway, but I would love to have more energy. It would be a good way for me to learn how I can help my patients'. Never one to turn down a sleep challenge and, at the same time, intrigued by this lady who seemed to be running on a different sort of energy but at the same time seemed to be incredibly motivated and committed to her work, I jumped at the opportunity. This is Karen's Sleep and Energy Story:

History:

Age: 49 years

Current sleep pattern: Goes to bed between 9.30 and 10pm. Wakes up at 4am, lies there waiting for alarm to go off at 4.30am when she rises from bed. Sleep initiation has always been a problem. Usually wakes several times during the night. Dreams a lot but very little dream recall.

Energy levels: Very buzzy in the morning. Exhausted in the afternoon. Finds it hard to do anything after 3pm.

Nutrition: Very little appetite in the morning so skips breakfast. Eats very little during the day but usually snacks on biscuits if they are 'lying around'. Eats healthy vegetarian meal in the evening.

Hydration: Maximum ½ litre water/day

Caffeine: 3-4 strong coffees, 1-2 cups of tea – all before 6am, strong latte on way to work, 3 espressos during day, 1-2 cups of tea in the afternoon.

Exercise: walking

Any other symptoms: premenstrual syndrome and monthly migraines which last 2-3 days.

Lifestyle: Karen spends the first 2hrs of the day meditating, writing and reading. Leaves for work at 7.30am. She begins work at 9am and works through the day without taking any breaks or stopping for lunch.

Personality: Karen drives herself very hard; she likes to do everything quickly and is very impatient. She walks and talks very quickly and hates the thought of anything slowing her down.

Goals: to have more sustainable energy, to improve sleep quality, to feel healthier in general.

To meet these goals Karen and I agreed on an initial action plan that would mainly involve using some Basic tools:

> Gradually cut down on caffeine (I asked Karen to think about how she would prefer to do this)
>
> Increase hydration to at least 1 litre of water/day
>
> Eat breakfast within an hour of rising
>
> Snack healthily between meals on energy bars, yoghurt, fruit, nuts and seeds

As these were quite significant changes that Karen needed to make, I really didn't want her to agree to make them unless she had really given them some thought. I also asked her to think about what she would stand to gain/lose by making these changes. To her great credit, Karen decided to spend some time reflecting on whether she really wanted to do embark on the programme. It took her very little time to decide that it really was a good idea. She very much wanted to take up the challenge so we embarked on the programme . . .

I asked Karen to keep me fully updated on her progress. What follows is a summary of the diary entries, text messages and emails that Karen sent to me in the weeks following her commencement on the programme:

Day 1: I have switched from coffee to tea. A bit worried about what will happen but have to keep reminding myself of why I am doing this.

Day 3: I am doing v well. Reassessing what tired means. Some interesting realisations about what I had thought was 'high energy'.

Day 7 (progress update sent by email):
I have made a number of changes:
I have increased my water intake by about 1litre – this is hard and I have to keep reminding myself to drink as I really don't like the taste of water.
I'm having breakfast (small amount of nutty muesli with milk, no sugar) around 6.30 –huge struggle initially but easier now.
Still having 5-6 cups of tea a day, am trying to replace with water, juice or herbal tea but still very drawn to caffeine.
Making myself have a snack at around 10-11am and if needed at around 1.30-2pm. I am having a light lunch while on the go.
I am starting to notice the difference:
I am falling asleep really easily (!) and waking up later at 5am so I'm definitely getting more sleep.
I am starting to feel hungrier (this is very new for me). I am eating more but not gaining weight.
Am checking how I really feel when I habitually think that I'm tired – have found that usually I am not actually tired – there is something else going on . . .
I have also found that I'm considerably slower in the mornings but actually

feeling more relaxed and less need to rush. I am consciously thinking about balance and trying to slow down.

I feel more mindful generally – with slower thoughts and a greater aware- ness of how my body is feeling but also what is going through my head. I find this very pleasant. I think I'm even becoming less reactionary; maybe even a little more tolerant and patient!!

In the afternoons, when in the past I would have felt so drained, my energy levels, although still lower than the mornings, don't feel so debilitating. I just don't feel drained the way I used to.

I realise that when I used to think I was 'tired', it was actually often the absence of that 'hyper' feeling. I had thought 'hyper' was my optimum level. This is still a bit of a challenge at times as part of me still has a sense that 'fast is best'. Anyway, I have begun to realise that I can get just as much done without needing to be quite so 'speedy'. I need to reflect some more on this, as I have always been this way and this is how most of my family tend to be. I am aware that this is quite a shift for me, psycho- logically, but something I've wanted to address for years.

Many thanks,

Karen

Ps I think I'm doing really well. Is this just the honeymoon period?

Day 9: All seems to be going well although i have a bit of a cold – runny nose and eyes – but feels as if my energy levels are balancing out and my body is going through a detox process… I am now using the caffeine-free tea bags with success – I don't seem to need the caffeine.

Meditation and life generally, including interaction with patients seems healthily slower, quieter, which I appreciate very very much. In meditation, especially, I have more of a sense of stillness and silence.

Day 11: I wanted to share with you my continuing progress . . .

I have been so aware the past few mornings, of coming in to work on the train, of walking in the 'herd' but feeling content to walk at the same speed as everyone else. I am so pleased! In the past I was always zig-zagging through the crowds and getting annoyed with people who seemed to be deliberately holding me back – it makes me laugh when I think of it now!! Also, I seem to be dreaming more and remembering my dreams – I'm really enjoying this as I like to know my dreams.

Most importantly, I am falling asleep effortlessly and this has been happening consistently for the past week. I am still tending to wake up during the night but whereas in the past I would have lain awake for an hour or more, I now seem to get back to sleep within a few minutes. Do you think I should stop looking at the clock each time I wake up – I think you may have mentioned this before?

Karen continues to make progress. She is still maintaining her positive changes. She still wakes at 5am but falls asleep easily, sleeps well and very rarely finds it hard to return to sleep if she does wake up. She now begins her day with energy instead of stumbling to the coffee machine as she once did. Karen has always been a lark – as are most of her family – and will always enjoy being an early riser. But now she can do so without the background worry of 'How am I going to make it through my day?' Her migraines are less frequent and less intense and debilitating. They now last less than 24hrs whereas in the past they would go on for up to 3 days.

In her most recent message to me Karen said

I am now trying to make sure I give myself a few moments between patients, even if I'm already running late. I also wanted to mention my new clarity in understanding what type of energy I need. This morning was a good example – I sensed something was not quite right energy-wise. Checked, and found physical energy levels very good and was able to sense that it was an emotional/spiritual energy issue that I needed to address in meditation. I am also more aware of my energy levels generally, of what's helpful and what's not.

Karen responded very quickly to my sleep programme. She is hoping to go on and use some of the power tools such as the optimal breathing technique and powernapping to further optimise the progress she has made to her sleep and energy levels. I believe that what helped enormously was her motivation – she had made a strong case for herself to stick with the programme by constantly reminding herself of her 'vision' and what she stood to gain by making the changes. This served as a reliable touchstone when she was faced with difficult choices. I also believe that Karen's meditation practice probably featured strongly in her rapid results as this seemed to give her a strong sense of self-awareness which enabled her to very quickly notice the early and subtle progress she was making.

CHAPTER 14

Frequently Asked Sleep Questions

The following are some of the questions that I am asked time and time again. All of the answers to these questions can be found in the body of Tired but Wired but I have included this chapter for quick and easy reference.

How much sleep do we need?

I am often asked this question and I try to guide my patients and clients towards developing flexibility and a greater self-awareness of their varying needs for sleep.

Our sleep requirements vary and the key is to become more attuned to what we need. We also need to remind ourselves that sleep is only one way of renewing our energy and in my experience, people who do not pay attention to other essential forms of energy renewal – nutrition, hydration, movement, relationships – are more likely to need more sleep.

However, to get a general idea of how much sleep you

should be getting, the work of Professor Jim Horne and other workers has described two types of sleep: *core* sleep versus *optional* sleep. Core sleep is the first three sleep cycles (the initial 4-5 hours of sleep) necessary for human beings to function properly. Optional sleep is the 'nice to have' sleep that we can reasonably do without – again, this is 4-5 hours.

I always wake up once or twice during the night. Is this normal?

It is completely normal to wake up during the night – I call this sleep 'elasticity' (page 40) and it is probably something we have evolved with as a survival mechanism to ensure that we could regularly emerge from sleep to check that our world was safe and we weren't going to be eaten by predators. Most people actually wake between 10-15 times per night but have no recollection of this as we enter a semi-conscious state called a hypnogogic trance. If you wake up, it is important to return to sleep effortlessly so avoid checking the time, putting the lights on and the key is to remain as sleepy as possible. Use the Optimal Breathing Technique (page 129) and its variations to help you slide back into sleep.

Why do I have problems sleeping on Sunday night?

Many people find it difficult to sleep on Sunday night and then feel the effects of poor sleep on Monday morning (sometimes referred to as 'weekend jet lag'). This inability to sleep on Sunday night could, in part, be a throwback to the school days when there might have been some lingering anxiety about unfinished homework. As you get older this translates into anxiety about what lies in the week ahead. A more likely reason for 'Sunday night syndrome' is that many people shift their sleep cycle forward at the weekends – going to bed later and rising later. They may also get more sleep than the weekday quota so that they are simply not as tired on Sunday night especially if they have had an afternoon nap after a heavy Sunday lunch.

I find it impossible to sleep during the day so can I learn how to power nap?

Anyone can learn how to power nap. The most important thing is to know what a power nap actually is and what it isn't. A power nap is *not* sleeping. It is 5 to 20 minutes of taking yourself to a deep state of relaxation in which you will be aware of your surroundings but you use your breathing as the focus to help you to relax. Use the technique on page 155 to help you to create a power napping technique that really works for you.

Can I learn how to sleep on planes?

I would encourage you to think in terms of relaxing on planes rather than actually sleeping. In this way, by taking the pressure off wanting to sleep you're more actually likely to do exactly that.

There are a few things that will also optimise the quality of your rest. These are: minimise caffeine before and during your flight, eat lightly, avoid surfing the movie channels and watching hours of in-flight entertainment, use aromatherapy oils such as lavender on your pulse points to induce sleepiness and relaxation, read a book that helps to relax your mind or listen to relaxing music, get as comfortable as you can – take off your shoes, loosen any tight clothing, make sure that you are warm, use comfortable eye masks to block out light, use the Optimal Breathing Technique (page 129) and variations to rest.

My job entails regular travel across time zones. Is there anything I can do to minimise jet lag?

Jet lag is what happens when the body's circadian timer and sleep/wake cycle is disrupted by crossing time zones. In theory, we should be better at adapting to going from east to west (creating a longer day) than by going from west to east (creating a shorter day) when sleeping becomes difficult and jet lag can take its toll. People respond differently to jet lag but there are some things that you can do to minimise its impact. These include following all of the healthy strategies outlined in the previous question on sleeping on planes.

I also find that practising meditation (page 173) while travelling really minimises fatigue and jet lag. I would recommend meditating for 10-20 minutes on takeoff and again for 10-20 minutes as the plane prepares to land.

Adjusting your sleep pattern a few days in advance can help. So if you are travelling east, start going to bed earlier and rising earlier to minimise the impact of the time difference. Getting some exposure to natural daylight when you arrive at your destination is also a good idea as is doing some gentle exercise and eating lightly and according to your destination's eating schedules

Melatonin is widely available in the United States and some people find that it helps to induce sleepiness and counteract jet lag. In the UK melatonin is not licensed as an over-the-counter medicine and according to the NHS, the benefits are inconclusive. So far the data both supports and challenges the use of melatonin in overcoming jet lag.

Homeopathic remedies containing a combination of Arnica,

Cocculus and Nux Vomica as well as other ingredients can also be used to naturally counteract the effects of jet lag.

Why do I wake up during the night worrying about things I need to do the next day?

Are you going to bed with a clean slate or, at least, a clear idea of what you need to do the next day? If not, get into the habit of writing an organised 'to do' list before you leave work or at least well before you get into bed (see page 106). Avoid working right up to the moment before you get into bed and *never* work in bed if you are a Sensitive sleeper. If worries stop you getting to sleep or getting back to sleep, use the Time to Worry technique on page 163.

I am getting 8 or 9 hrs of sleep every night so why am I so tired?

Remember, sleep is only one way of recovering and renewing your energy so take a look at the Energy Pyramid (page 74) and think about how you are renewing your energy on all of the levels – physical, mental, emotional and spiritual. Are there any other habits you should be paying attention to other than sleep?

Also, your tiredness could be due to poor quality sleep – is your caffeine intake high or do you use a lot of other stimulants such as nicotine or alcohol? Are you drinking enough water? Is there enough rest in your day? Do you eat breakfast first thing in the morning – not eating breakfast can often cause sluggishness first thing in the morning. Sleeping too much can also be related to illness or depression so if the tiredness persists you may need to see discuss this with your doctor.

Why are my dreams so vivid?

Everyone dreams but not everyone remembers his or her dreams. Are you very creative but not expressing your creativity? Have your dreams become more vivid recently and has this coincided with you being under a lot of stress lately? If so, can you find an outlet for your stress – talk or write about it? Don't forget to minimise stimulants such as caffeine – this can make your dreams much more disturbing. Take a look at the Power Tools (IV) section of the Sleep Toolkit for exercises that will help you to manage and understand your dreams.

Why do I keep waking up at 3am?

We go into our shallowest stages of sleep around this time so if the conditions aren't perfect for sleep we are more likely to wake. Non-ideal conditions would include caffeine, alcohol, and other stimulants and your worries and problems. You are also more likely to wake in the early hours if you suffer from depression or anxiety.

Try to steer clear of stimulants, avoid checking the time when you wake up, try to remain as sleepy as possible, avoid putting lights on, use the OBT (page 141) and/or Count Yourself to Sleep or Surf the Breath techniques to steer yourself back into sleep. If necessary, use the Time to Worry Tool (page 163) to keep worries and anxieties away from your sleep.

Why can't I remember my dreams?

Not everyone does remember their dreams. Dreams are most likely to occur during the hypnagogic or hypnopompic trance states in REM sleep when sleep is at its shallowest. You are more likely to remember your dreams if the information from your dream is 'transferred' into your conscious mind and working memory'. If it remains in your subconscious memory, you will just have a vague sense of it and it will begin to recede as soon as you start to recall it. If you want to get better at remembering your dreams then keep a pad and pencil by your bed and write them down as soon as you wake up.

How can I get to sleep after my night shift?

The challenge for the night shift worker lies in the fact that their sleep drive will be working in opposition to the circadian timer or sleep clock. Simply put, this means that you will be feeling sleepy when your body rhythms are telling you to be awake and alert. To key to optimising sleep after working a night shift is to build up enough of a sleep drive (i.e. to be sleepy enough) to sleep when you come off your shift. This means that during your shift you should manage your energy carefully – minimise stimulants and try to avoid caffeine for at least 3-4 hours before you will be getting into bed, avoid having a heavy, high-fat meal during your shift, eat small amounts regularly every 2hrs or so throughout your shift to maintain alertness and stabilise your blood sugar levels (and optimise melatonin production for sleep), try to keep active and move regularly during your shift. When you come off your shift have a small snack before sleeping such as a bowl of cereal and milk or a milky non-caffeinated drink, use sleep-inducing aromatherapy oils such as lavender in your bedroom, use a white noise machine or fan to minimise external sounds, use black out curtains or a comfortable eye mask to minimise light, set a wake-up alarm and avoid checking the time if you do wake before your alarm. Later in the day use Replacement Naps (page 153) to top up your sleep if you wake up ahead of your alarm going off. Try to build some activity into your day when you wake up – 20-30 minutes of brisk walking – and stay well-hydrated.

Does sex help you to sleep?

Another popular question! Human beings can really be quite different in this regard; while some people might find the rush of endorphins and serotonin positively relaxing and soporific, others might find it stimulating and definitely not sleep-inducing.

I wake up at the slightest noise. Is there anything I can do about this?

First of all check that your stimulant (caffeine, alcohol, nicotine) intake is low as they promote light sleep. Then use some form of white noise or a fan to minimise interruptions from external sounds. See the Useful Resources section for information on white noise machines.

Is it good to read to get to sleep?

Absolutely! But the key is to keep it light, philosophical, uplifting and not too stimulating or involving plots that you *have* to get to the end of (I tend to read books like this on holiday).

How can I get back to sleep when my children wake me up during the night?

First of all, avoid checking the time. Try to stay as sleepy as possible, keep the lights low if you can. Use the OBT (page 141) and variations to return to sleep.

My brain is buzzing when I get back from work late. What can I do to get to sleep?

Make sure that you have a clear idea of what you need to do at work the next day – ideally you would write a list before you leave the office. Allow yourself time to wind-down – even if it means delaying getting in to bed by half an hour or so. Keep the emphasis on doing everything SLOOOOOWLY and use the OBT as you go about your wind down. Switch off your mobile phone and BlackBerry. Go through the Pre-Sleep Yoga or Letting Go exercise for at least 10 minutes before getting into bed. Use the OBT with the Sleep Counting (page 143) or Surf the Breath (page 145) variations to help you fall asleep.

I live on my own and have recently moved into a new flat but I'm finding it very hard to get to sleep at night.

Do you feel safe in your new home? And if not, what can you do to make yourself feel safe? Apart from the obvious things like ensuring your flat is secure, what can you do to create a more comforting, nurturing and peaceful environment? Think about smells (candles, aromatherapy oils), flowers, colours, lighting, pictures. Use the OBT (page 141) combined with the Gratitude (page 168) or Optimism (page 165) exercises to help ease you into sleep.

I think I sleep better when I'm not sharing my bed with my partner. Is this normal?

This is very normal and while some human beings love sharing their 'caves' with their partners, others find that their sleep is much more disrupted when they share their bed. In my sleep practice, I find much marital discord that arises from exactly this – particularly if a Martini sleeper shares a bed with a Sensitive sleeper. The solution lies in compromise and communication – can you negotiate sleeping separately if you are going through a particularly bad patch with your sleep or if you have a big event the next day and really *need uninterrupted* sleep? If you can't do this, can you use white noise to minimise your partner's nocturnal noises? You may need to investigate a larger bed or a good quality mattress that is singly sprung.

My baby is 3 weeks old and I love being a mum but I'm exhausted because of lack of sleep. Is there anything I can do about this?

It is really important to pay attention to all of the factors that influence your energy and that are within your control – eat healthily following the nutritional guidelines in the Basic Toolkit (page 113), stay well hydrated and minimise caffeine and alcohol so that whatever sleep you do get is of good quality. Try to nap and power nap (page 152) whenever baby does even if it means letting go of some of the household chores. Can you negotiate with your partner, relative or friend some interrupted time so that you can take a replacement nap (page 153) every now and then? Remember, it will get better *and* it may be some small consolation to know that your ability to cope with sleep deprivation actually improves as a result of the hormonal and emotional changes that occur along with pregnancy and birth.

My baby is 11 months old but I'm still not sleeping well. Can I do anything about this?

Many new parents find that this happens after the birth of their child. The important thing is to rebuild your connection with your sleep. Take a look at the Nuts and Bolts Tools (in particular the wind down routines) on page 97 to see whether there are some small changes that will make a big difference. Also, have you got back to exercising regularly? If not, try to do a little exercise every day – even 30 minutes of brisk walking per day will help.

Finally, take a look at the Letting Go exercises (page 149) or Pre-Sleep Yoga routine to help you relax before bed.

I can't stop moving my legs and it stops me getting to sleep. What can I do about it?

You may be suffering from restless legs syndrome (RLS) (see page 59). This can be related to an iron deficiency that can be shown by a blood test so it might be worth a trip to your doctor. Relaxation techniques, and in particular the Pre-Sleep Yoga routine, (page 147) and the Legs up the Wall exercise with progressive muscle relaxation (page 150) can help to relieve the symptoms.

How can I stop myself feeling sleepy when I drive?

The best thing to do is to open all of the windows and put the radio on loud until you can stop at a service station. When you get there, close your eyes and power nap (page 152) for 15–20 minutes to ease your tiredness and sharpen up your concentration. For an added boost, and if you have several hours of driving ahead of you, try a having a cup of coffee *before* doing your powernap.

Why am I so tired in the mornings? I continually press the snooze button for at least an hour before I'm ready to get out of bed.

This is a pattern that I often notice with my patients and clients who are stuck in a fatigue cycle (page 52). To break the cycle, start eating breakfast *within 30-45 minutes of rising* (page 113), snack healthily between meals, stay well hydrated and minimise caffeine and alcohol.

Is there anything I can do to stop myself snoring during the night?

This can be caused by excess abdominal weight and is also associated with having a thick-set neck (collar size 17 inches or more). Make sure that you are well hydrated, minimise alcohol, use eucalyptus aromatherapy oils on your pillow to aid breathing. In the long term regular exercise and yoga, with an emphasis on breathing techniques, can be particularly helpful.

I find it hard to get to sleep if I've got a big event on the next day? Is there anything I can do about this?

This is often related to a fear of 'if I don't sleep I won't perform at my best'. I try to reassure my clients by reminding them that we are well equipped to deal with the odd night of poor sleep and, in fact, research suggests that it doesn't affect performance significantly. I also encourage my clients to think in terms of 'rest' rather than 'sleep' and to tell themselves that they can potentially recover more energy by resting efficiently than by tossing and turning and trying to sleep. Using the Time to Worry (page 163) exercise followed by the Legs up the Wall exercise (page 147) might also be beneficial. Have you got a Perfect Bedtime Story (page 165) that you can use to get you to sleep?

Sometimes as I am dropping off to sleep my legs suddenly jerk and twitch and I feel as if I am falling.

This can happen as the body and mind 'unload' the stress of the day. Try to practise the Pre-Sleep Yoga routine (page 147) or Legs up the Wall exercise for 10–15 minutes before getting in to bed.

I'm coming off my sleeping tablets and I'm scared that I won't be able to sleep.

First of all, never come off your medication suddenly. Make sure that you discuss this with your doctor who will agree with you a programme of gradually reducing your dosage of sleeping tablets. While you have been on the tablets, they have been controlling your internal sleep chemistry so your body may experience some disruption while it tries to find its own balance again. This is analogous to someone who has broken their leg and then removes the cast – they are going to feel a bit weak and wobbly to start off with until the muscles regain their full strength. There are a few things that you can do to help yourself get back to full strength:

1. Be prepared for a few bad nights – treat your sleep like the British weather.
2. Pay attention to all of the other aspects of your energy to minimise fatigue. Revisit the Basic Tools section in the Sleep Toolkit (page 112).

3. Use powernapping to minimise fatigue if you do have a
   bad night. But remember, nap for no more than 15-20
   minutes.
4. Hold on to your vision to help you stay motivated.
5. Support yourself with natural and complimentary
   therapies such as homeopathy, reflexology, acupuncture or
   reflexology.

My ten year old daughter struggles every night to fall sleep and she is often tired and irritable during the day. Can I use the Sleep Toolkit to solve her problems or is it just for adults?

Children really need their sleep — it is absolutely vital for the process of learning and their physical growth. This is particularly the case in today's world when many children's days are packed with school and after-school activities.

The Toolkit can definitely be put to good use with children. Starting with the Nuts and Bolts tools, make sure she winds down before bed and doesn't spend too much time at the computer or watching TV. Ideally she should have at least an hour or so free from electronic equipment (TV, mobile phone, computer or electronic games) before she gets into bed. Is she getting enough exercise during the day? Is her diet reasonably free of stimulants and sugary snacks? She should take a daily multivitamin tablet to ensure that she is getting all of her micronutrients — especially the ones vital for sleep. Make sure that her bedtime reading is light and not over-stimulating. A bedtime milky drink might help her to relax. Use lavender oils in her bath or white noise if she is particularly sensitive to sounds. Try introducing her to the Pre-Bedtime Yoga routine (page 147).

Talk to her about what is going on at school and whether

there is anything that is particularly worrying her. Try to listen without jumping in with an instant solution and explore with her how you can best support her if there is something on her mind. Some children respond very well to writing down things that they don't want to verbalise. If this is the case she may find it helpful to keep a journal.

I've found that children respond particularly well to the Optimism and Gratitude exercises (pages 165 and 168). Spend a little time doing this with her in the evening as part of her bedtime routine. She could even use a journal to record the 'ten good things that happened in my day . . .' Finally, recent research shows that children who are taught meditation are calm and confident at school and suffer less stress and sleep problems. You could start by showing her how to meditate for 1 minute and gradually building up to 5 minutes. Ideally she could do this before she gets into bed or even sitting up in bed using a word of her choice such as 'calm' or 'peace'.

THE TOOLKIT MADE EASY

A refresher guide of the Sleep Toolkit with corresponding page numbers where longer descriptions can be found.

Nuts and Bolts Tools:

These are simple and practical tools to really get you started thinking about your sleep and the steps you can take to improve it.

Wind down routines   (p. 97)

What are your sleep rituals and how can you practice more positive ones?

Your ideal sleep environment   (p.100)

What do you need to do to make your sleep environment feel just right for you?

Timing   (p. 103)

Are you a lark or an owl? What is the best time for you to go to bed?

Bed comfort   (p. 105)
Pillows, linens, blankets etc

Switch it off!   (p. 106)
No phones, laptops, BlackBerries in bed! Turn the TV off!

Time management   (p. 106)
Get on top of your to-do list before you go to bed.

Stop checking the time!   (p. 108)
Do you really need to know the time when you wake up
during the night?

Basic Tools:

These four tools are the foundation to a healthy, well-balanced
lifestyle and are also instrumental in helping you achieve the
deep, restorative sleep you desire.

Nutrition: 6 Steps to Good Sleep   (p. 113)
The most important nutritional strategies to follow for good
sleep.

Stimulants   (p. 118)
The effect of caffeine and alcohol on your sleep.

Hydration   (p. 122)
How drinking water affects your sleep.

Exercise and Movement   (p. 123)
How exercise can help you sleep better and how much you
should be doing.

The Power Tools

The Power Tools take practice and discipline but can really lead to big shifts in behaviour and improve the quality of your sleep. As I've said before make a commitment and try something for 21 days to start seeing change.

POWER TOOLS I – BREATHING:

The Optimal Breathing Technique (OBT)   (p. 132)
A simple but powerful breathing technique that will transform your sleep.

POWER TOOLS II:

Count yourself to sleep   (p. 143)
Combining the OBT and a simple counting technique to put you to sleep.

Surfing the breath   (p. 145)
A gentle method to lull you to sleep that combines the OBT with the waves and your imagination.

Pre-sleep yoga   (p. 147)
A simple yoga routine to set you up for peaceful sleep.

Letting go   (p. 149)
The power tool to help you let go of a stressful day.

The power of napping   (p. 152)
Napping tools to recoup energy during the day and enhance the quality of your sleep.

POWER TOOLS III – MIND POWER:

Time to worry   (p. 163)

The tool to use if worrying gets in the way of good sleep.

The perfect bedtime story   (p. 165)

    -The optimism exercise   (p. 165)
    -The gratitude exercise   (p. 168)
    -Your own perfect bedtime story   (p. 170)

Now I lay me down to sleep . . .   (p. 172)

The tools for ending the day on the right note and setting up deep nourishing sleep.

Meditation   (p. 173)

The ultimate power tool for creating deep, rejuvenating sleep.

POWER TOOLS (IV):

Stream of consciousness dream journaling   (p. 190)

Keeping a dream journal for more peaceful sleep.

Chaos narrative dream journaling   (p. 191)

Dealing with overwhelming dreams.

Lion posture   (p. 193)

Get it off your chest!

FURTHER READING

Chapter 1

James Gleick, *Faster,* Little Brown and Company: London, 1999

Claudio Stampi et al, *Why We Nap. Evolution, Chronobiology and Functions of Polyphasic and Ultrashort Sleep,* Birkhäuser: Boston, 1992

Chapter 2

Antonio Damasio, *The Feeling of What Happens,* William Heinemann: London: 1999

Daniel L Schacter, *How the Mind Forgets and Remembers. The Seven Sins of Memory,* Souvenir Press: London, 2001

Jim Horne, *Why We Sleep: The Function of Sleep in Humans and Other Mammals.* Oxford University Press: Oxford, 1988

Jim Horne, *Sleepfaring. A Journey Through the Science of Sleep,* Oxford University Press: Oxford, 2006

Rita Carter, *Mapping the Mind.* Weidenfeld & Nicolson: London, 1998

Rita Carter, *Consciousness*. Weidenfeld & Nicolson: London, 2002

William C Dement, *The Promise of Sleep: The Scientific Connection Between Health, Happiness and a Good Night's Sleep,* Macmillan: London, 2001

Chapter 3

Colin Espie, *Overcoming Insomnia and Sleep Problems,* Robinson: London, 2006

Helen Kennerley, *Overcoming Anxiety,* Constable & Robinson: London, 1997

Michael Krugman, *The Insomnia Solution,* Warner Books: New York, 2005

Richard O'Connor, *Undoing Depression,* Souvenir Press: London, 2010

Simon Wessely, Matthew Hotopf and Michael Sharpe, *Chronic Fatigue and its Syndromes,* Oxford University Press: Oxford, 1999

Chapter 4

Alyssa Abbey, *Stop Making Excuses and Start Living With Energy,* Capstone: London, 2008

Anthony Robbins, *Unlimited Power,* Pocket Books: London 2001

Bill Ford, *High Energy Habits,* Pocket Books: London, 2002

Jim Loehr and Tony Schwartz, *The Power of Full Engagement,* The Free Press: London, 2003

William Collinge, *Vital Energy,* Thorsons: London, 1998

Chapter 6

The Mind Gym, *Give Me Time,* Time Warner Books: London, 2006

Chapter 7

Patrick Holford, *Optimum Nutrition for the Mind*, Piatkus: London, 2003

Jane Clarke, *Body Foods for Busy People*, McBooks Press: London, 2006

Jackie Habgood, *The Hay Diet Made Easy*, Souvenir Press: London, 1997

Khush Mark, *Fat Doesn't Make You Fat*, Effervescent Life: London, 2008

Chapter 8

H. David Coulter, *Anatomy of Hatha Yoga*, Body and Breath Inc: USA, 2001

Ilchi Lee, *Brain Respiration*, Healing Society Inc: USA, 2002

Paul Wilson, *Calm for Life*, Penguin Books: London, 2000

Chapter 9

Shakti Gawain, *Creative Visualization*, New World Library: USA, 1995

The Sivananda Yoga Centre, *The New Book of Yoga*, Ebury Press: London, 2000

Desmond Dunne, *Yoga Made Easy*, Souvenir Press: London, 1999

Chapter 10

HH Dalai Lama & Howard C Cutler, *The Art of Happiness*, Hodder and Stoughton: London, 1998

Daniel Goleman, *Emotional Intelligence*, Bloomsbury: London, 1996

Dean Ornish and Stephan Bodian, *Meditation for Dummies*, Wiley Publishing Inc: NJ, 2006

Eckhart Tolle, *The Power of Now*, Hodder and Stoughton: London, 2001

Gillian Butler and Tony Hope, *Manage Your Mind*, Oxford University Press: London, 1995

John Purkiss, *All in the Mind*, John Purkiss: London, 2004

Jon Kabat-Zinn, *Wherever You Go, There You Are, Mindfulness Meditation for Everyday Life*, Piatkus: London, 1994

Martin E P Seligman, *Learned Optimism*. Vintage Books: London, 2006

Martin E P Seligman, *Authentic Happiness*, Nicholas Brealey Publishing: London, 2003

William Bloom, *Feeling Safe. How to be Strong and Positive in a Changing World*, Piatkus 2002

Chapter 11

Allison Price, *Writing From the Source*, Thorsons: London, 1999

Linda Caine and Robin Royston, *Out of the Dark*, Bantam Press: 2003

Julia Cameron, *The Artist's Way*, Pan Books: 1995

Julia Cameron, *The Artist's Way Workbook*, Souvenir Press: London, 2007

Louise DeSalvo, *Writing as a Way of Healing*, The Women's Press Ltd: London, 1999

Robin Royston and Annie Humphries, *The Hidden Power of Dreams*, Bantam Press: 2006

Brian Alman, Peter Lambrou, *Self Hypnosis: The Complete Guide to Better Health and Self-Change*, Souvenir Press: London, 1993

USEFUL INFORMATION

British organisations with specialist knowledge in sleep therapies and complementary fields, and further information on alternative medicines and accredited practitioners.

Use these resources as a springboard for investigating the different forms of guidance available to you to improve your sleep.

UK Sleep Hospitals, Sleep Societies and Helpline

Capio Nightingale Hospital
Capio Nightingale Hospital
11–19 Lisson Grove,
Marylebone
London
NW1 6SH
www.nightingalehospital.co.uk

British Sleep Society
PO Box 247,
Colne, Huntingdon,
PE28 3UZ,
England, UK
http://www.sleeping.org.uk

The London Sleep Centre
137 Harley Street
London
W1G 6BF
Email:
info@londonsleepcentre.com
Website:
http://www.londonsleepcentre.com/

Sleep Matters Helpline
(Medical Advisory Service)
PO Box 3087
LONDON
W4 4ZP
Email:
info@medicaladvisoryservice.org.uk

Helpline: 0208 994 9874
Website:
http://www.medicaladvisory
service.org.uk/

British Snoring and Sleep
Apnoea Association
Castle Court
41 London Road
Surrey
RH2 9RJ
E-mail:
info@britishsnoring.co.uk

The Sleep Council
High Corn Mill
Chapel Hill
Skipton
North Yorks
BD23 1NL
Email:
info@sleepcouncil.org.uk
Website:
www.sleepcouncil.com

Sleep Apnea Trust
The Sleep Apnoea Trust
12a Bakers Piece
Kingston Blount
Oxon
OX39 4SW
United Kingdom
http://www.sleep-apnoea-
trust.org

The Edinburgh Sleep Centre
13 Heriot Row
Edinburgh
EH3 6HP
0131 524 9730
http://www.edinburghsleep
centre.com/

Sleep Scotland
8 Hope Park Square
Edinburgh
EH8 9NW
Scotland
Tel: 0131 651 1392
http://www.sleepscotland.org/
sleepc.php

Dept of Sleep Medicine
The Royal Infirmary of
Edinburgh
51 Little France Crescent
Old Dalkeith Road
Edinburgh
EH16 4SA
http://www.sleep.scot.nhs.uk/

Narcolepsy Association UK
(UKAN)
PO Box 13842
Penicuik
EH26 8WX
Telephone: 0845 4500394
Email: info@narcolepsy.org.uk
Website:www.narcolepsy.org.uk

Alternative Medicine

British Complementary
Medicine Association
(BCMA),
P.O. Box 5122,
Bournemouth,
BH8 0WG
Tel: 0845 345 5977
http://www.bcma.co.uk

Association of Natural
Medicine
27 Braintree Road
Witham
Essex CM8 2DD
Telephone/Fax: 01376 502762
http://www.associationnatural
medicine.co.uk/

British Homeopathic
Association
Hahnemann House
29 Park Street West
Luton
LU1 3BE
Tel: 01582 408675
http://www.britishhomeo
pathic.org/

Alternative Health UK
Directory
http://www.alternativehealth.
co.uk/

Therapy and Counselling

British Association for
Counselling and
Psychotherapy
BACP House,
15 St John's Business Park,
Lutterworth,
Leicestershire LE17 4HB
Tel: 01455 883300
http://www.bacp.co.uk/

British Holistic Medical
Association (BHMA)
PO Box 371
Bridgwater
Somerset
TA6 9BG
Tel: 01278 722 000
http://bhma.org

Federation of Holistic
Therapists (FHT)
18 Shakespeare Business
Centre
Hathaway Close
Eastleigh
Hampshire
SO50 4SR
Tel – 0844 875 20 22
http://www.fht.org.uk

Society of Holistic
Practitioners
4 Craigpark
Glasgow
G31 2NA
Tel: 0141 554 5808
http://www.societyofholistic
practitioners.com/

Yoga and Meditation

BWY Central Office,
British Wheel of Yoga,
25 Jermyn Street,
Sleaford,
Lincolnshire,
NG34 7RU
Tel: 01529 306851
http://www.bwy.org.uk/

Yoga Scotland
http://www.yogascotland.org.
uk/

London Meditation Centre
www.londonmeditationcentre.
com

Cindy Cooper, Mindfulness
Teacher and Trainer in
London, cindy@mindfulness-
london.org.uk
Fully accredited by the

Centre for Mindfulness
Research and Practice.
http://www.bangor.ac.uk/
mindfulness

Aromatherapy

Aromatherapy Trade Council
PO Box 387
Ipswich
IP2 9AN
Tel: 01473 603630
http:// www.a-t-c.org.uk

White Noise Machines

Michelle Knights (01694
723900)
www.whitenoisemachine.
co.uk

Spa Relaxation Sound Machine
www.homedics.co.uk

Reflexology

Association of Reflexologists
5 Fore Street,
Taunton,
Somerset,
TA1 1HX.
01823 351010
http://www.aor.org.uk

Massage

General Council for Massage
Therapies
27 Old Gloucester Street
London
WC1N 3XX
Tel: 0870 850 4452
http://www.gcmt.org.uk

Association of Holistic
Biodynamic Massage
Therapists
42 Catherine Street
Cambridge
CB1 3AW
Tel: 01223 240815
http://www.ahbmt.org/

Acupuncture

British Acupuncture Council
63 Jeddo Road
London
W12 9HQ
Tel: 020 8735 0400
www.acupuncture.org.uk

British Medical Acupuncture
Society (BMAS)
Royal London
Homoeopathic Hospital
60 Great Ormond St
London WC1N 3HR
Tel: 020 7713 9437
http://www.medical-acupuncture.
co.uk/

ACKNOWLEDGEMENTS

I want to thank all of the people in my life who made the writing of this book possible:

To all of my patients and clients over the years who have truly brought the theory to life for me.

To Louise Orpin for spinning her magical spider web. Kerry-Lyn Stanton-Downes for her support and ideas. Dr Andrew Norman for the clever introduction. Shona Hood for critique, listening skills and babysitting. Lisa Lewisohn for encouragement and taking a huge load off my shoulders. To all of my friends for kind words and positive energy. To all at Souvenir Press, especially Ernest Hecht for taking a punt and Lara Mathers for her calm guidance.

A special thank you to Andrew Kwok who made it safe for me to not sleep.

To my wonderful parents without whom this would never have been possible. You have given me the vital ingredients that have kept me (relatively) balanced and made me who I am.

Finally, to my little family, Peter and Maya. Peter, you've been my partner in this every step of the way. I thank you for your patience and belief and for enduring yet another of my obsessions. Maya Nirvana, as always, my inspiration and lucky star. You are an incredible little being. Thank you for understanding when I have had no choice but to hibernate and write.